ISNR Research Foundation
1925 Francisco Blvd. E. #12
San Rafael, CA 94901
cynthia@isnr.org

ISBN: 978-0-9846085-1-5

v. 2 Update Design: Cynthia Kerson, PhD

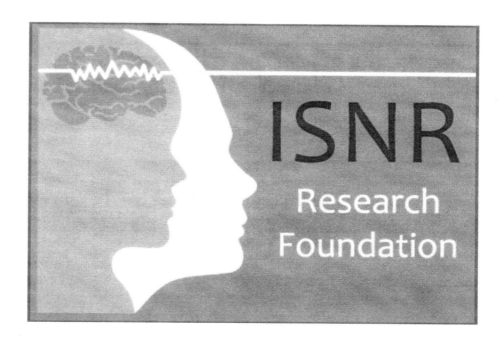

Contact the authors:
D. Corydon Hammond, PhD: d.c.hammond@utah.edu
Jay Gunkelman, QEEGD: qeegjay@sbcglobal.com

Table of Contents

Introduction

The purpose of this book is to provide a practical, introductory training manual on the art of artifacting quantitative EEG data. We begin by explaining how to record an EEG in a way that minimizes artifactual data in the record. We then define and illustrate the majority of the artifacts that are encountered in clinical practice. The next section of the book is unique. You will be provided with an extensive practicum exercise in identifying common artifacts from actual raw EEG data from several different patients. After analyzing each page of raw data, you can thumb to the end of the book and learn which of the epochs on that page we found acceptable, and what artifacts were identified in each second of the data.

It is our hope that this book and practicum exercise will foster practical skill development, providing you with some basic competence in identifying artifacts prior to receiving training in quantitative EEG. We recommend, however, that as you begin gathering qEEG data that you arrange to work wi.th a very experienced consultant initially who can assist you in identifying artifacts until you reach a level where you are in virtually unanimous agreement with the consultant on artifacts that are present in raw EEG data. When there is not a convenient local consultant available, such tutoring can be done over the telephone or through the Web so that you may both examine the same epochs simultaneously. It is also valuable to study some of the EEG atlases that are available (e.g., Goldensohn, Legatt, Koszer, &Wolf, 1998).

All royalties from the sale of this book have been donated to the Society for Neurofeedback and Research. It is our small way of expressing thanks to our many respected colleagues and friends, while at the same time seeking to provide funds that will enable the society to provide further training in quantitative EEG and neurofeedback to clinicians. We acknowledge our appreciation to the Q-Metrx service for providing examples of several artifacts. This volume is lovingly dedicated to our children, Matthew and Erin Hammond, and Vaughn Gunkelman.

Preparation and EEG Recording to Minimize Artifacts

An artifact refers to a modification of the EEG tracing that is due to an extracerebral source. Artifacts are inevitably present in every EEG, like crabgrass in the lawn, but they may obscure EEG activity and lead to misinterpretations when the EEG is transformed into topographic displays. Artifacting refers to the careful examination of the raw EEG data and the post-hoc removal of artifacts prior to qEEG analysis.

The wise clinician does not simply screen out EEG segments with artifacts in them. The number of artifacts may be tremendously reduced by skillful work in recording the EEG. This begins by educating the patient about major sources of artifacts. For instance, you can have him or her generate artifacts while viewing the computer screen as they tense their neck, move their tongue (e.g., saying, "La, la, la," or "Tom Thumb"), tense their jaw and forehead, move their head, blink their eyes, and make vertical and then horizontal eye movements under closed lids. If the patient is sniffling at all, he or she may also be asked to sniff their nose a couple of times. The clinician may even record the patient doing each of these at the beginning of the EEG for later reference. Placing large cotton balls over the closed eyes, and then putting a snug sleep mask on over the cotton balls also assists in reducing eye movement. Alternatively, the clinician may gently place a finger over the closed eyelids to discourage eye movement. We always rest a towel behind the patient's neck so that the back of the head and posterior electrodes do not touch the chair. We also instruct the patient,

"Gently, slowly close your eyes. Relax your face now. Let your jaw hang down limply, with your lips parted, your mouth comfortably open and teeth not touching, your face relaxed, and your tongue seeming to just float quietly in space, without touching your teeth or the roof of your mouth, and swallow as infrequently as you can."

Quality recordings are also obtained by carefully checking impedances. Electrode impedances should always be below 5000 Ohms. Ear electrode impedances may be reduced by avoiding placing electrodes over pierced holes, and by applying electrodes to the rear of the earlobe, where the skin is less weathered. Excess paste should be removed so as to not conduct signals from larger areas. We further recommend not allowing inter-electrode impedance differences of more than 500-1000 Ohms. The closer the inter-electrode impedance levels were, the more reliable the recording.

Something that has not been emphasized enough, but that we consider to be vitally important, is to balance the impedance level between the linked ears. This means that the impedance level of each ear compared to the vertex ground electrode should be as perfectly balanced in readings as possible. This is essential if one is to avoid obtaining spurious interhemispheric differences. Another equally important point, and yet one that we have never seen before in print, is that the impedances should be balanced as perfectly as possible between homologous (interhemispheric) electrodes. This is of considerable importance in light of research on frontal and parietal hemispheric asymmetries in depression and anxiety (e.g., Davidson, 1998a, 1998b; Heller et al., 1995, 1997) or panic disorder (Wiedemann, et al., 1999). Neurofeedback not uncommonly focuses on interhemispheric, homologous sites. For example, Rosenfeld

(1997) created a protocol for normalizing the frontal alpha asymmetry associated with depression. In clinical practice using such neurofeedback applications, we likewise consider it just as important to have close to perfectly balanced impedance levels between comparable interhemispheric electrodes.

As an aid in securing good impedances, we ask patients to shampoo their hair 3 times on the day of the recording, not to use hair conditioners or shampoo containing conditioners, and to use no hair spray. In patients with bald, shiny heads, we use an alcohol wipe with a light scrubbing of NuPrep prior to putting on an ElecroCap. Portable telephones should also be turned off prior to EEG recording or neurofeedback work.

Before recording, it can be helpful to ask patients to produce various artifacts. This helps to impress upon patients the sensitivity of the recoding and need to follow instructions, and it also allows the clinician to document the appearance of various artifacts in individual patients. Thus, you may ask patients with their eyes closed to look to the right, look to the left, to look up, look down, blink, move their tongue up and down against the back of their teeth and roof of the mouth, move their tongue back and forth (or to say, "La, la, la," or "Lilt"), and to tense the jaw. These may even be recorded at the beginning of the record, and pausing the EEG to note the epochs associated with each artifact that was voluntarily produced. A double-sided preliminary screening form that Dr. Hammond created for his own use, and on which space is provided to note such things, is reproduced in Appendix.

We like to have the patient's eyes closed for 30 seconds before starting to record to avoid state changes. Prior to recording, it is also advisable to briefly observe the EEG data, pausing it occasionally and looking for major artifacts. Thus, if you observe EMG (muscle tension) in the right temporal area or forehead, you may ask the patient to relax his or her face and jaw, while continuing to observe data until the artifact is no longer present. Unfortunately, we can't always eliminate all artifacts through this kind of skillful preparation for the recording. Sometimes, no matter how hard you try, you cannot get a patient to eliminate all the tension in his forehead, jaw, or neck, which may subsequently be reflected in frontal, temporal, or occipital channels. In such cases, one must simply take this into account in interpreting the results and note it in a report.

Once recording has begun, it is also valuable to pause the EEG recording whenever you see an artifact beginning to appear in the data (e.g., muscle tension), or when you begin to see the amplitude and definition of the EEG decline, indicating that the patient is entering stage 1 sleep. Thus, as you pause the recording, you may also ask the patient if he or she is drowsy, although the patient may not be subjectively aware of this yet. Nonetheless, you can ask patients to move their arms and legs, wiggle their thumbs, and instruct them to be certain to remain relaxed, but nonetheless alert and awake. When pausing a recording to control artifacts, remember that positive reinforcement for compliance is far superior to criticism or providing negative feedback. There is an old saying in research and statistics classes: Garbage in, garbage out." For a quantitative EEG to provide a valid, meaningful, and reliable assessment of the patient, the epochs that are accepted for analysis must be as artifact-free as possible. As we have indicated, this is accomplished first of all through careful preparation and data acquisition. Afterwards, the clinician must skillfully artifact the data, ascertaining with each epoch, "Is this data fact, or artifact?"

Common Artifacts

EMG (Muscle) Artifact

EMG artifact will occur in the higher alpha and beta range. The higher the amplitude with increasing frequency (e.g., especially over 23 Hz), the more likely it is that muscle artifact is imitating beta activity, although muscle artifact may include frequencies as low as 13 Hz (Lee & Buchsbaum, 1987; O'Donnell, et al., 1974; Oken, 1986; Willis, et al., 1993). EMG artifact should particularly be suspected when it seems to appear on one or two channels, since genuine EEG will usually occur on several channels. EMG artifacts are particularly seen at T3 and T4, but are also frequently seen in frontal areas, and sometimes at T5 and T6, and in the occipital area due to muscle tension in the neck. It is possible to find EMG artifacts on any channel. When a patient with a cold sniffles, this will also produce a burst of muscle artifact (most likely in the Fp1 and Fp2 channels), sometimes followed by a slow wave (so that it may even resemble a spike and wave complex). Parkinson's patients who have a head tremor will often produce a rhythmic, theta frequency artifact that will most likely be seen in occipital channels. In patients with tics or involuntary movements of hands or legs, these can be monitored with an extra EMG channel to assist in distinguishing their influence (Klass, 1995). One may also inquire of patients with temporal EMG artifact to determine if they wear dentures. Sometimes removing the dentures may reduce artifact.

In qEEGs muscle activity was found to increase the percent power in beta above 24 Hz in the channels 01, 02, P3, P4, T5, and T6 in one study (Willis et al., 1993). The authors found that the posterior region of the head was stable for frequencies up to 24 Hz whether muscle artifact was being generated or not. But, above 24 Hz, muscle artifact altered recorded EEG activity at virtually all sites. Beta activity below 24 Hz was stable in the posterior regions (01,02, P3, P4, T5, T6) whether muscle activity was present or not, and, therefore, they concluded that these electrode sites would be most suitable for the study of beta activity in quantitative EEG. Your current authors would argue that with good monitoring and recording all sites are suitable candidates for study.

When tension is seen in the record, pause the recording and assist the patient in reducing muscle tension in the problematic area(s) through suggestions to relax that area, allow the lips to remain open, or through gently massaging the skin nearby. Occipital EMG activity may be associated with having the head bent backwards or posterior electrodes touching the chair. Correcting the placement of the head may eliminate this EMG activity. When it is not possible to eliminate all EMG from the record, qEEG reporting systems that provide 1 Hz topographic maps and relative power spectra for each electrode site are valuable in further evaluating the location of EMG activity at different hertz levels (e.g., 15-16 Hz versus 24+ Hertz). This detailed documentation and analysis allows the real EEG to be differentiated from EMG artifact. An example of EMG artifact on channels T3 and T4 is seen in Figure 1 to the left.

Movement Artifacts

Body movement, head movement, or movement of the electrode wires can create artifacts. Therefore, it is important to encourage the patient to remain perfectly still, including not to move his or her head, and for the clinician to be observant for this and to note precisely when movement occurs. Movement artifact can particularly be a problem in children or in patients with tremors or movement disorders. Importantly, keep a rolled or folded towel behind the patient's neck so that the head and posterior electrodes do not press against the back of the chair. However, the size of the folded towel should be such that it does not position the head awkwardly in a manner that will encourage muscle tension in the neck or head. The towel should also not disturb the electrodes in the cap, but merely stabilize the head. Movement artifact may also be minimized by assuring that the patient is in a comfortable position and then by pausing the EEG every 3-4 minutes to allow the patient to wiggle and readjust his or her posture, which at the same time helps to control drowsiness. However, once again, allow the eyes to remain closed for 30 seconds before beginning to record again to avoid state transitions. A patient with a Parkinson's head tremor will tend to produce theta frequency waves in the occipital area (Westmoreland et al., 1973). In recording patients with Parkinson's or a tic, it is helpful to have a supplementary EMG channel.

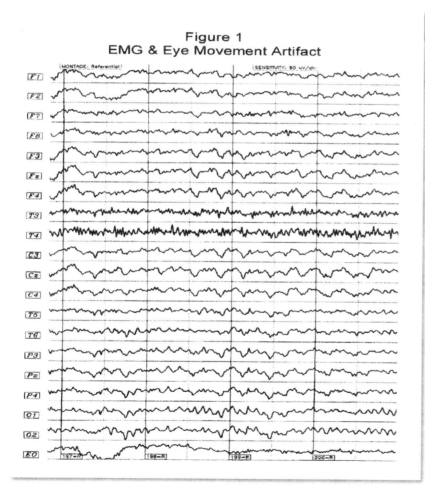

Figure 1
EMG & Eye Movement Artifact

Eye Blink & Eye Movement Artifacts

Having an eye movement channel is very important in identifying eye movements. The over 100 milliwatt difference between the aqueous and vitreous humor is the source of the eye dipole. The active electrode may be placed between the eyes, just above eye level, with a reference electrode just below the outer edge of the eye, close to the bone. Although eye blinks will usually be seen fairly symmetrically at Fp1 and Fp2, a separate eye channel assures identification of blinks or eye movements. Eye blinks are typified by the sharp contour of the wave, often with a triangular shape, and their occurrence in frontal leads. If a wave is an eye blink, it will generally be most

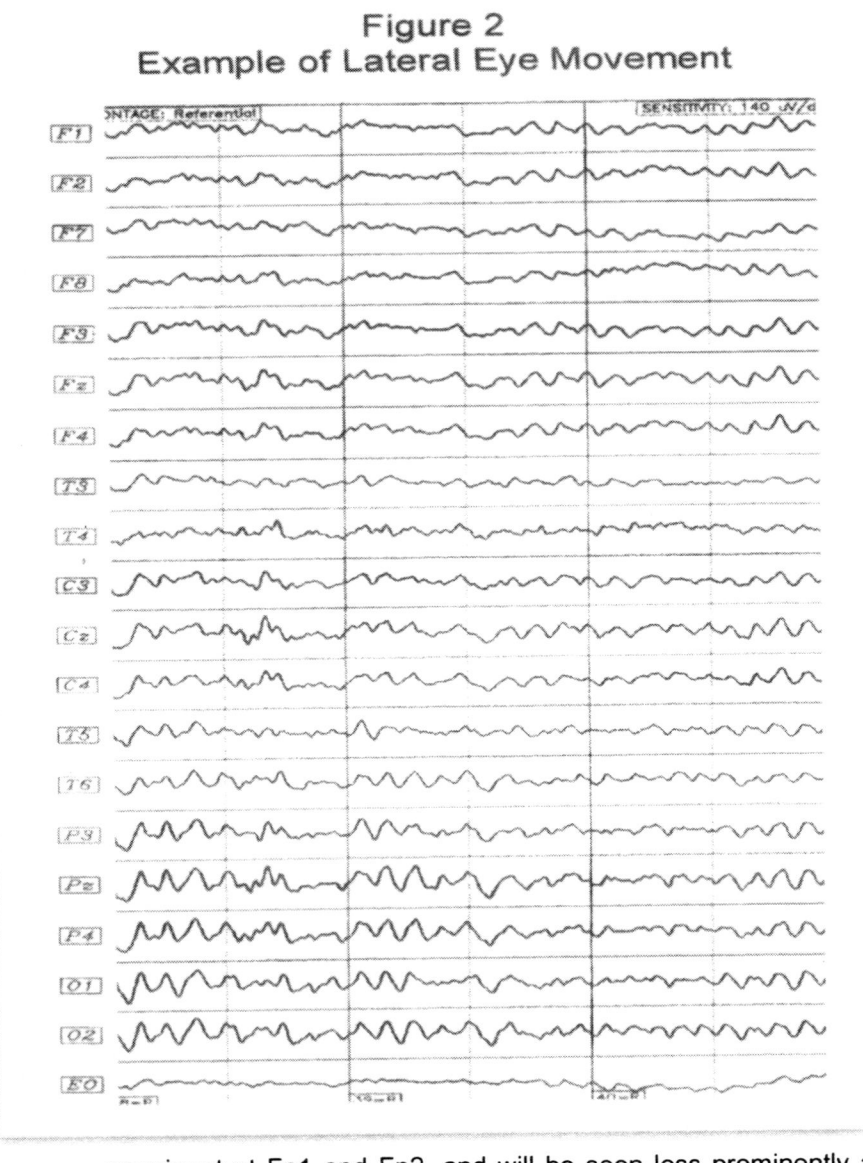

Figure 2
Example of Lateral Eye Movement

and F4 than it was at the frontal poles. This artifact can be mistaken or frontal intermittent rhythmic delta activity (FIRDA). An example of vertical eye movement is seen in the first second of data in Figure 1.

It must also be noted that effects from eye movements may also influence electrodes into the central and temporal areas. When examined on a longitudinal sequential montage, vertical eye movement will be seen as a downward deflection of the Fp1-F3 and Fp2-F4 channels. Lateral eye movements will also be detected by watching for phase reversal on F7-F8 (as illustrated in Figure 2), and in a longitudinal sequential montage, it will produce movement toward Fp1 or Fp2 in Fp1F7 and Fp2-F8 channels respectively. If two supplementary channels are available, both vertical and horizontal movement may be measured separately. Eyelid flutter, particularly in anxious patients, will appear as a frontal rhythmic activity in the range of 5-10 Hz. It is only by observing the patient carefully during the recording that one can distinguish this from genuine frontal theta or alpha. Similarly, observing the patient will help to identify slow eye movements beneath closed eyelids, which are observed in the F7 and F8 channels and are an early sign of drowsiness (which will be discussed below).

Fisch (1991) provided the following insights into eye movement artifact, which reinforce the value of examining raw data with different montages, as we will discuss shortly:

"The frontal origin of eye movement artifacts may remain unclear in referential montages, particularly those using ear electrodes which

prominent at Fp1 and Fp2, and will be seen less prominently at F3

may be contaminated by eye movements. Repetitive eye movements may mimic cerebral rhythms; slowly repetitive eye movements may closely resemble bilaterally synchronous frontal slow waves, and repetitive eye movements associated with lid flutter during eye closure may cause frontal rhythms of about 10Hz. As a general rule, it is best to assume that activity in the alpha frequency range localized to the frontopolar head regions is eye movement artifact until proven otherwise. (P. 111)."

A more jagged appearing artifact may be caused by rapid eye movements, and eye movement artifact may also include muscle artifact. Thus, for example, you may see a lateral rectus spike which was caused by a muscle artifact preceding a lateral eye movement. Such an artifact must not be confused with spike and wave activity.

EKG and Pulse Artifact

EKG or cardioballistic artifacts tend to be seen across all or most channels (although often with greater prominence in temporal areas) at the heart rate's frequency of about 1/second. EKG artifacts in particular are more likely to occur in patients who are overweight and who have thick or large and muscled necks. This artifact will be detected with greatest precision when a separate EKG channel is recorded so that the clinician may definitively see when the pulse occurs, and can then look across the other channels to determine if the timing of the EKG coincides with activity across a variety of channels. Pulse artifacts are common and may be difficult to eliminate. They are more likely to be seen in the temporal area and may result from an electrode which contained an air bubble or that is being moved with the pulsation of an adjacent blood vessel. Filling an electrode more fully may eliminate the artifact by eliminating the

bubble. It has also been suggested (Mowery, 1962) that having the patient turn his or her head to the right may help eliminate EKG artifact.

The occurrence of EKG artifact in the recording of the EEG may be an unavoidable cardioballistic effect, but it may also be due to an impedance imbalance between the ear electrodes (which will reduce the out-of-phase cancellation of the inverse EKG signal between the two ears). Therefore, the first thing to do when this is noticed prior to data recording is to double check the ear impedance and equalize them again if needed. If the impedance of both ears are equal (and low enough for good recording) and the EKG persists, switching the display to a Laplacian or a sequential montage will minimize the appearance of the EKG signal. However, cardioballistics are unavoidable in some individuals in referential montages. An example of EKG artifact may be seen in Figure 9 on page 21.

The millivolt (MV) level of the EKG signal is orders of magnitude stronger than the microvolt (uV) signal of the EEG. In referential recordings, such as linked ears, the reference electrode is run in parallel to all 24 channels, thus reducing the common mode rejection ratio proportionate to the number of parallel channels and allowing the strong field effect from the cardiac generators to be seen more readily. For the times when the EKG is unavoidable, knowing the signature in the qEEG of the artifact helps in interpretation to be able to "read around" the artifact. The periodicity of the QRS complex (the spike portion of the EKG waveform) gives the qEEG topographic maps an apparent voltage at the frequency of the repetition rate for the heart beat. The faster frequency components of the EKG may be seen in rare circumstances in topographic spectral plotting, although this is rare since transient events are not well displayed in the qEEG due to averaging.

When EKG-related artifact cannot be eliminated, the practitioner should be aware that although it occurs with a frequency of about once a second, nonetheless its waveform has other frequency components and so it may influence not only delta, but also possibly alpha and even beta. Furthermore, since the wave will be common to other electrodes, it will artificially increase coherence.

Glossokinetic Artifacts &Swallowing

The tongue forms a dipole with the tip of the tongue being negative in relation to its base. Thus, just as eye movements can create electrical activity because of the dipole of the eye, tongue movements result in potential changes that may likewise produce artifact. Glossokinetic artifacts are most likely to resemble delta, slow wave activity. An example is seen in Figure 3. Rapid tongue movements in the antero-posterior direction are the most likely to produce this artifact. Therefore, prior to beginning a recording EEG technologists may ask patients to say, "La-la-la," "Lilt," "Tom Thumb," and also to swallow to evaluate how this artifact may look for the individual patient, and compare it with what is seen later in their recording. This is valuable because only about 27% of patients have been found to produce a detectable glossokinetic artifact (Jaffe & Brown, 1983). It is most likely to be prominent in frontotemporal channels. Without awareness that it is artifactual, this could be misinterpreted as frontal intermittent rhythmic delta activity (FIRDA). Once again, observation of the patient during recording will be invaluable in identifying this kind of artifact. If the patient has dystonia with orofacial dyskinesia, habitual tongue movements, or a tic, we are likely to see this artifact. Instructions to "keep the mouth slightly open, lips parted, tongue floating peacefully in space without moving, and trying not to swallow very often," will help to minimize this artifact.

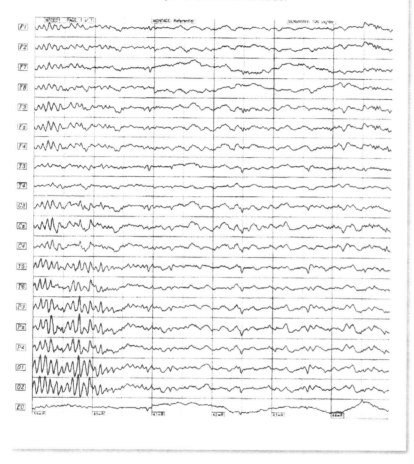

Figure 3
Example of Glossokinetic Artifact

Another intraoral artifact identified by Milnarich et al. (1957) is a sharp discharge stemming from dissimilar metals in the mouth. Once again, this is more prominent in frontotemporal channels and it resembles a static discharge or spike-and-wave complex.

Artifacts Associated With Drowsiness

Drowsiness has been found to be associated with a variety of different EEG patterns (Santamaria & Chiappa, 1987), some of which can be misperceived as being abnormalities (e.g., epileptiform sharp waves) unless the pattern of drowsiness is recognized. Similarly, in quantitative EEG analyses, if the clinician does not recognize drowsiness in the record and subsequently does not reject those epochs it may lead to the false positive conclusion that there is excess theta activity or centrofrontal alpha when, in fact, it is not present in the eyes closed and awake condition. Rhythmic and bilateral, notch-topped theta in the mid-temporal area is usually regarded as representing drowsiness (Duffy et al., 1989). Frontal theta or sometimes alpha, followed a few seconds later by a decrease in posterior alpha activity, should be considered a sign of early drowsiness.

Hughes (1994) explained:

"Another problem is to differentiate abnormal theta from similar activity that can appear in very early drowsiness. The latter activity can also represent a considerable problem for the electroencephalographer since it may be the only drowsy pattern to appear simultaneously with alpha activity, which usually designates a waking stage. Clearly, normal frontal theta of drowsiness can be seen, while the alpha is present, but its proper interpretation usually depends on other EEG signs of drowsiness that should appear within 5 to 10 seconds, such as the decrease in alpha (p. 117)."

A large proportion of people are sleep-deprived (Dement, 1999). Therefore, we particularly recommend that prior to recording you should ask, "How many hours of sleep have you had each of the last two nights." "How would you rate your degree of alertness right now, as 'rested,' 'slightly tired,' 'moderately fatigued,' or 'extremely fatigued or drowsy.'" This information can assist you in predicting how focused you need to be in maintaining vigilance.

As already mentioned, patients cannot be relied upon to necessarily recognize when they are drowsy. It can, however, usually be detected by noticing when the EEG begins to lose definition and flatten out. It may also be distinguished by seeing slow, asymmetrical, roving eye movements (e.g., at F7 and F8). In association with such drowsiness, the record may show vertex sharp waves, spindles, and generalized sharp waves, but can sometimes include POSTS, midline theta, and bursts (a group of waves appearing and disappearing abruptly that is distinguishable from the background activity) of increased amplitude activity with paroxysmal sharp morphology slow waves in children (hypnagogic hypersynchrony), and bursts of beta (13-30 Hz, but usually 14-16 Hz) occurring maximally in the fronto-centro-temporal areas (see Bartel et al., 1995, for good examples of these patterns). In drowsiness, alpha rhythm will usually attenuate or even disappear. Alpha will also spread anteriorly for 1-10 second periods with a concurrent decrease in the amplitude (and frequency) of occipital alpha (Santamaria & Chiappa, 1987). An example of this is seen in Figure 4 where alpha is present in the frontal, temporal and central areas, while it was not prominent earlier in the recording. Seconds later, posterior alpha begins to diminish and the entire recording begins to flatten out as drowsiness increases.

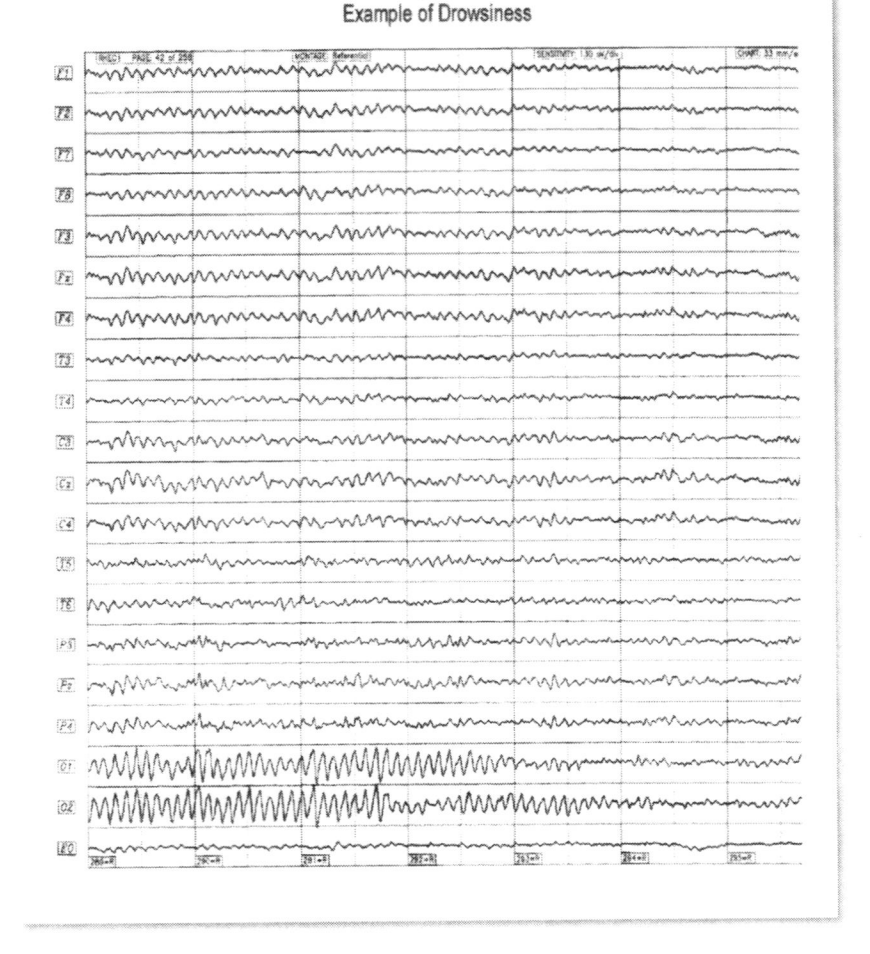

Figure 4
Example of Drowsiness

Sweat or Electrodermal Artifact

Very large, undulating, pendulous, and very slow waves (e.g., 1/4 wave/second) that are usually present in more than one channel are typical of sweat artifacts. They are most likely to occur in the frontal and temporal areas, and the amplitude appears inconsistent with cerebral activity. This artifact can be distinguished from eye rolls because it will usually not be maximal at F7 and F8 and it will not show the phase reversal but characterizes horizontal eye movements.

The example of raw data seen in Figure 5 illustrates perspiration artifact as it is seen in different montages. Note the general slow activity seen maximally at C3.

Very slow waves (lasting more than 2 seconds in duration) "should never be considered unequivocal evidence of an underling cerebral dysfunction unless accompanied by other changes such as slowing in the theta frequency range, or amplitude changes in the alpha and beta range" (Fisch, 1991, p. 116). However, Fisch (1991) notes that sweat artifact accompanied by generalized background slowing should alert the clinician to inquire about hypoglycemia.

A preventative is to keep the recording room cool or provide a gentle fan to reduce perspiration, especially when using a tight, elastic electrode cap. Nervous and anxious patients may produce this artifact independent of the room temperature due to the eccrine sweat gland's sympathetic nervous system innervation.

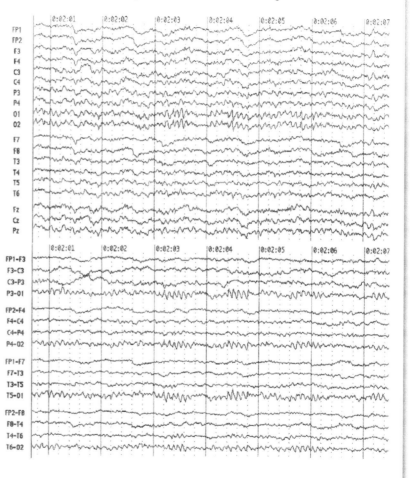

Figure 5
Example of Sweat Artifact in Different Montages

Salt Bridge

This is an artifact that occurs because of the excessive use of electrode paste or from sweating or applying the cap to a wet head so that the overflow builds a bridge between two electrodes. It is most prone to occur in using electrode caps as contrasted with individually applied electrodes, although it may be seen in any electrode system. In switching montages, a salt bridge will be apparent between the two involved channels because it will create a relatively flat tracing when placed in the same channel sequentially or bipolarly. Figure 6 on page 19 illustrates the "salt bridge" or electrical short between the 01 and 02 electrodes in a referential montage, and then seen as a flat line in a sequential montage.

Breach Rhythm

Breach rhythm refers to an artifact in which the amplitude is larger in a region of one hemisphere compared with the other due to a skull defect (e.g., burr holes, craniotomy and/or skull fracture). The skull attenuates and laterally diffuses activity, especially faster activity. The defect in the skull magnifies or exaggerates the activity that is present so that it appears higher in voltage. The resulting higher amplitude on the affected location might resemble spikes, but should not be misinterpreted as epileptiform discharges. Prescreening questions about any previous head injuries or head surgeries may alert the clinician to be particularly watchful for this artifact.

Electrode Artifact

When one electrode is found to deviate, it may not be well connected. Recheck the impedance. When this is not identified ahead of time or during artifacting, one electrode on the map will generally be lit up with what is popularly called the "comet effect," alerting the clinician to recheck the raw EEG. An electrode "pop," however, affects more than one channel and is usually seen as an abrupt deflection that may occur from time to time as the impedance becomes impaired. It may come from the ground or reference electrodes if seen on all channels, or from a wire or electrode jack that has an impaired connection and needs replacement. Remember, it is okay to pause in data collection to recheck impedances. When there is any question about good connections, they may also be rechecked after data collection is completed. Figure 7 on page 20 provides an example of an electrode artifact on the T4 channel.

Event Related Potentials

Event-related potentials are typically intermixed with EEG rhythms. The general rule for rejecting a transient is to reject the EEG epoch when the transients are 50% greater than the the background activity and represent a "change in kind" from the ongoing activity. Although their effect in averaged data may be minimal, they will increase variability and reduce reliability. Therefore, a conservative approach to epoch selection would dictate the exclusion of a transient if it meets the two rules just presented. An example of a transient is seen in the first two seconds of Figure 8 on page 17.

Artifacts from Environmental Sources

The clinician should be aware that environmental influences may also create artifacts in either qEEG data or during neurofeedback, such as cellular telephones that have not been turned off, lightening, a walkie-talkie being operated nearby, hospital infusion or dialysis pumps, and even earthquakes. These field effects are reduced through good skin preparation so that impedances are low and balanced.

Artifacts Due to Medication Effects

Medications may significantly alter EEG activity. For example, benzodiazepine tranquilizers commonly produce excess beta activity, lithium will usually produce a slowing of alpha and of delta, and some antidepressants will decrease alpha activity. It is beyond the scope of this volume to detail the diverse medication effects. The reader is referred to the volume *Drugs and Their Effects on Neurodiagnostics* (American Society of Electroneurodiagnostic Technologists, 1997), Glaze (1990), and Bauer and Bauer (1999).

The Role of Re-Montaging in Artifacting

Remontaging is a technique of algebraically recombining previously recorded referential EEG data into new montages not previously recorded. This technique gives the digital EEG an advantage over the older paper EEG recording technique. Remontaging gives the EEG a new perspective, independent of the original reference point.

A contaminated reference will give an artifactually distorted view of the EEG data. If the reference point is not a neutral point, the EEG which is used to form the qEEG images and statistical tables will form a distorted image due to the contaminated reference. As an example of this, if the ear reference is contaminated due to excessive temporal alpha, any surface site containing this alpha will not show it fully due to the common mode rejection, and any site without alpha will show the alpha, which is in the reference. Similarly, a temporal/frontal discharge or temporal EMG contaminating ear references may distort the EEG as seen in a referential montage and resulting topographic maps.

Remontaging is useful in evaluating the qEEG, which may have contaminated reference points. Since the EEG signal is the difference between the reference and the active electrode, any contamination of the reference will create artifactually distorted images, as well as artifactually distorted numerical data. Unless the perspective of the reference is changed, there will be an inability to see whether the images and numerical data are real or if the data are distorted.

The American Academy of Neurology (AAN) and the EEG and Clinical Neuroscience Society recommend remontaging all qEEG data to evaluate the neutrality of the reference site, and to give some perspective on which data more truly represents the actual EEG voltage and frequency distribution, absent the distortion of the reference site. As an example, if the ear references have contamination due to excessive temporal alpha (as may sometimes be seen in chronic migraine), any area without significant alpha, such as the frontal lobe, will display alpha due to the differential amplifier's normal function. Figure 10 on page 22 provides an example of how such false frontal alpha may appear before and after remontaging.

Frontal alpha may be seen in clinical cases such as OCD, depression, anxiety, and even attentional problems. However, if the qEEG data shows frontal alpha that is artifactually created due to the temporal alpha contamination, a false clinical impression may be made. Unfortunately, all current databases have linked ear norms. Though remontaging is needed to see whether the data is an accurate reflection of the brain's function, we all are currently limited with the normative database's inaccurate data in cases where distortions are noted. A remontagable database will be one of the next big steps in the field of qEEG.

Remontaging may also be used to reduce some artifacts. One example of this is the cardioballistic artifact (seen in Figure 9, p 21), and another is 60 Hz "line" interference. Both of these artifacts share a commonality, the highly coherent and phase locked "synchronous" nature of their waveform across all channels. These "field-effect" artifacts, the electrical field disturbance of the heart's currents, and the electrical field of the line currents (60 Hz generally, 50 Hz in some countries), both are virtually eliminated with remontaging to a weighted average "Laplacian" montage, or even to a sequential montage ("bipolar"). Similarly, EKG artifacts may be removed through using a weighted average montage. Figure 9 (page 21) illustrates how remontaging eliminates field effects.

Different montages provide different angles or windows for examining our data. All montages have their own distinctive limitations, and thus it is recommended that several different montages be utilized during the process of artifacting and in interpreting qEEG data. For example, Dr. Bill Hudspeth points out that weighted average and Hjorth montages do not really remove waveforms that are common across the head, so as to reveal unique waveforms at each electrode. Rather, they only remove common features in the local region (neighbors) surrounding each active electrode. Thus, when anterior and posterior electrodes show alpha activities that can be removed with either the weighted average or Hjorth montages, one cannot infer that the anterior alpha originated in posterior regions. The proof, or disproof, for such an hypothesis must be based upon correlations or coherences between the source (e.g., posterior, temporal) and destination (anterior) electrodes. When those relationships are low (insignificant), there is no empirical basis for a contamination from the posterior or temporal electrodes. Parsimony would then suggest that the anterior alpha arose from the sensorimotor system.

Once again, all references and montages have their own advantages and limitations. Ear references are not as good in identifying temporal lobe pathology, but they display drowsiness well. A Cz reference seems to better facilitate examination of the frontal alpha asymmetry which is found in depression, but is not a good reference if the patient is drowsy.

A coronal or transverse sequential ("bipolar") montage is very nice in examining slow wave focus and phase reversal, for example, with lateral eye movements or to localize a seizure "spike." Likewise, an average reference can be very sensitive in examining local problems, but not be as powerful with a more global problem. We must bear in mind that there is a potential problem with all montages, but most especially if someone relies on only one.

Figure 8
Example of a Transient

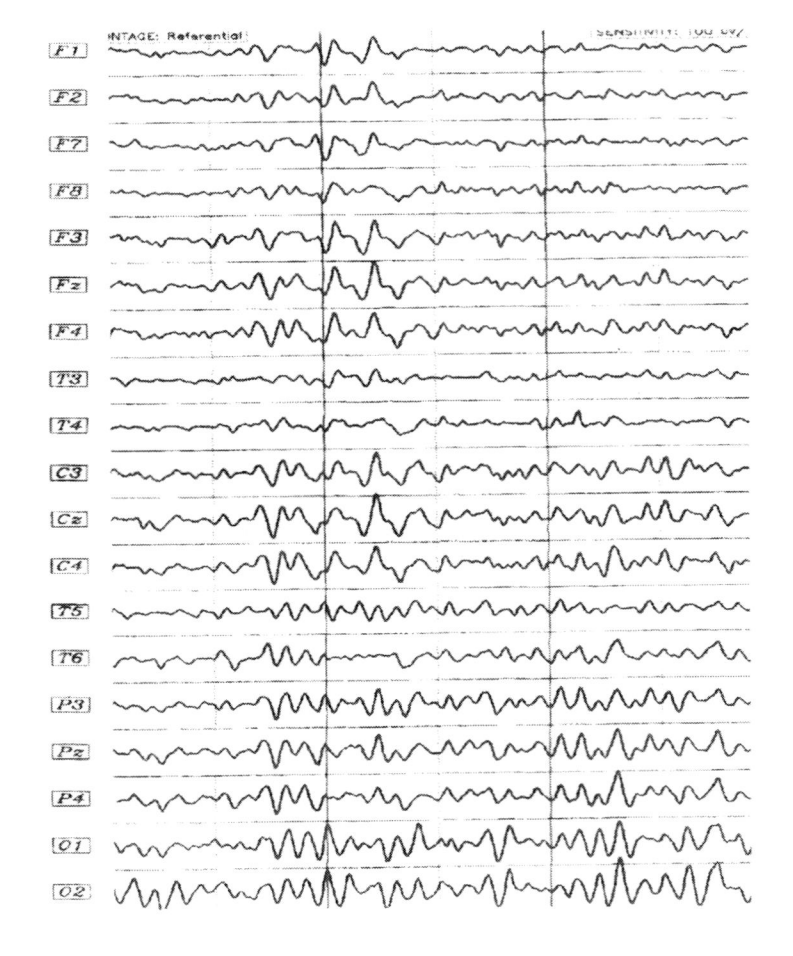

Figure 6
Example of Salt Bridge Artifact in Different Montages

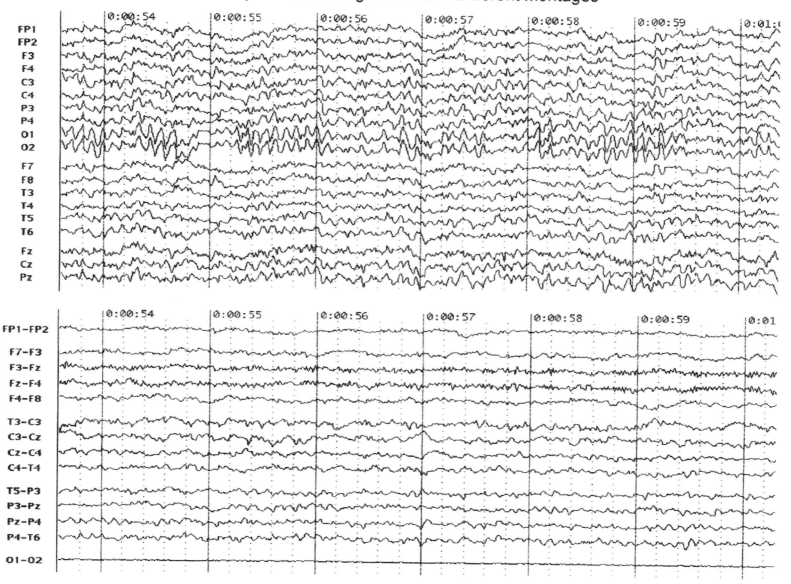

Figure 7
Example of an Electrode Artifact

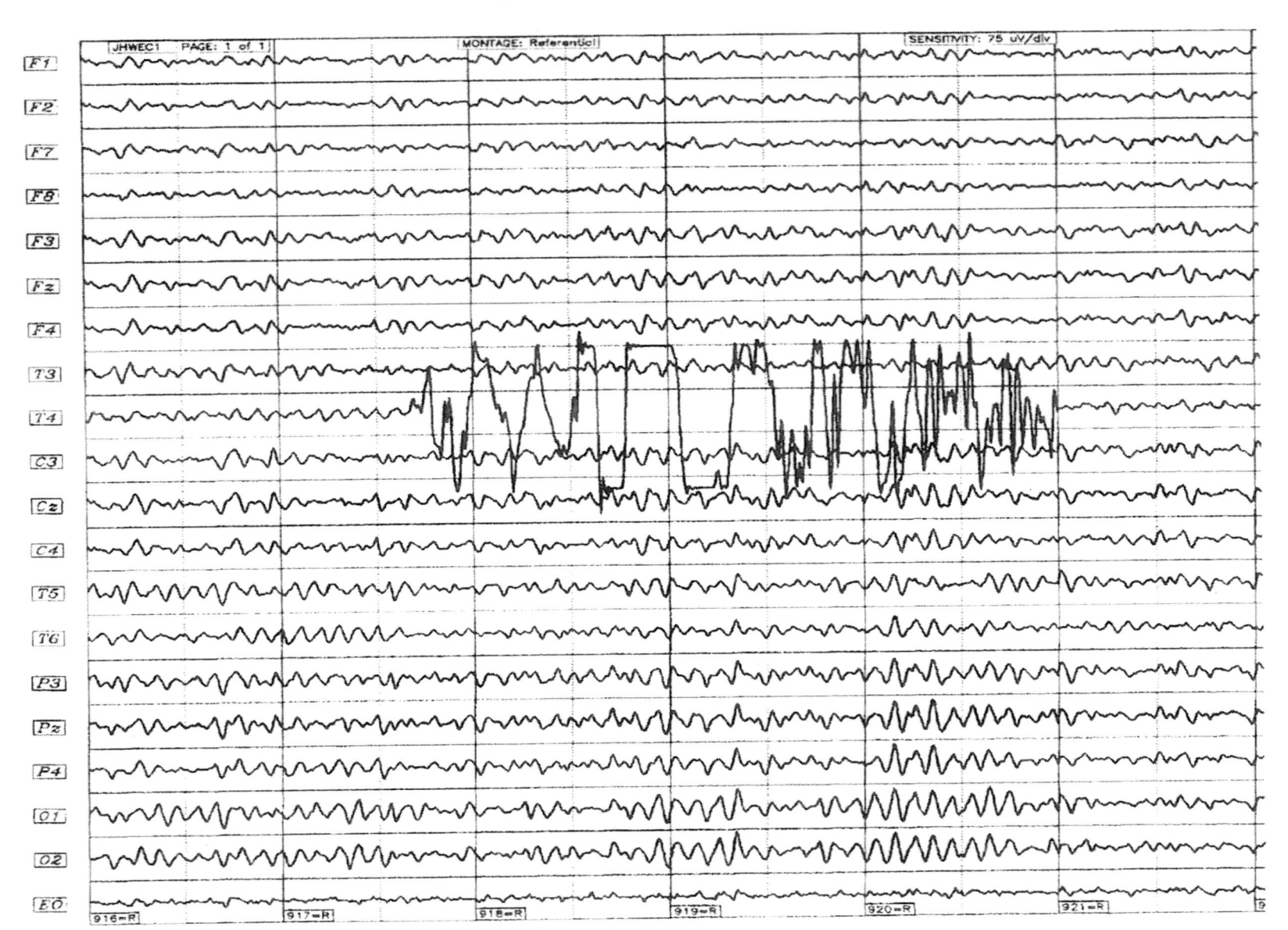

Figure 9
Examples of EKG Artifact with Two Referencing Methods

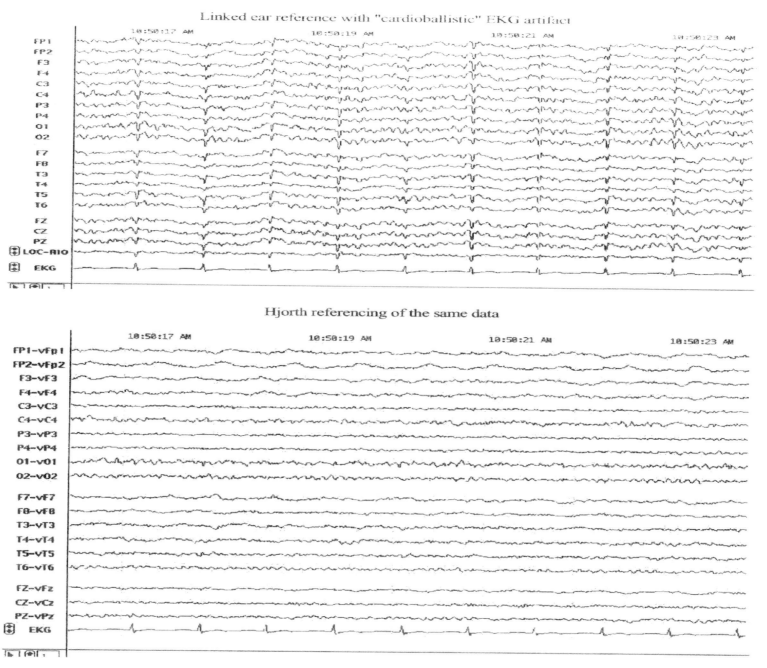

Linked ear reference with "cardioballistic" EKG artifact

Hjorth referencing of the same data

Figure 10
Examples of Differences in Frontal Alpha Before and After Re-montaging
To view these images in color: visit www.isnr.org/AOAPg20Fig10.html

Linked Ears / Eyes Closed   Hjorth Re-montage

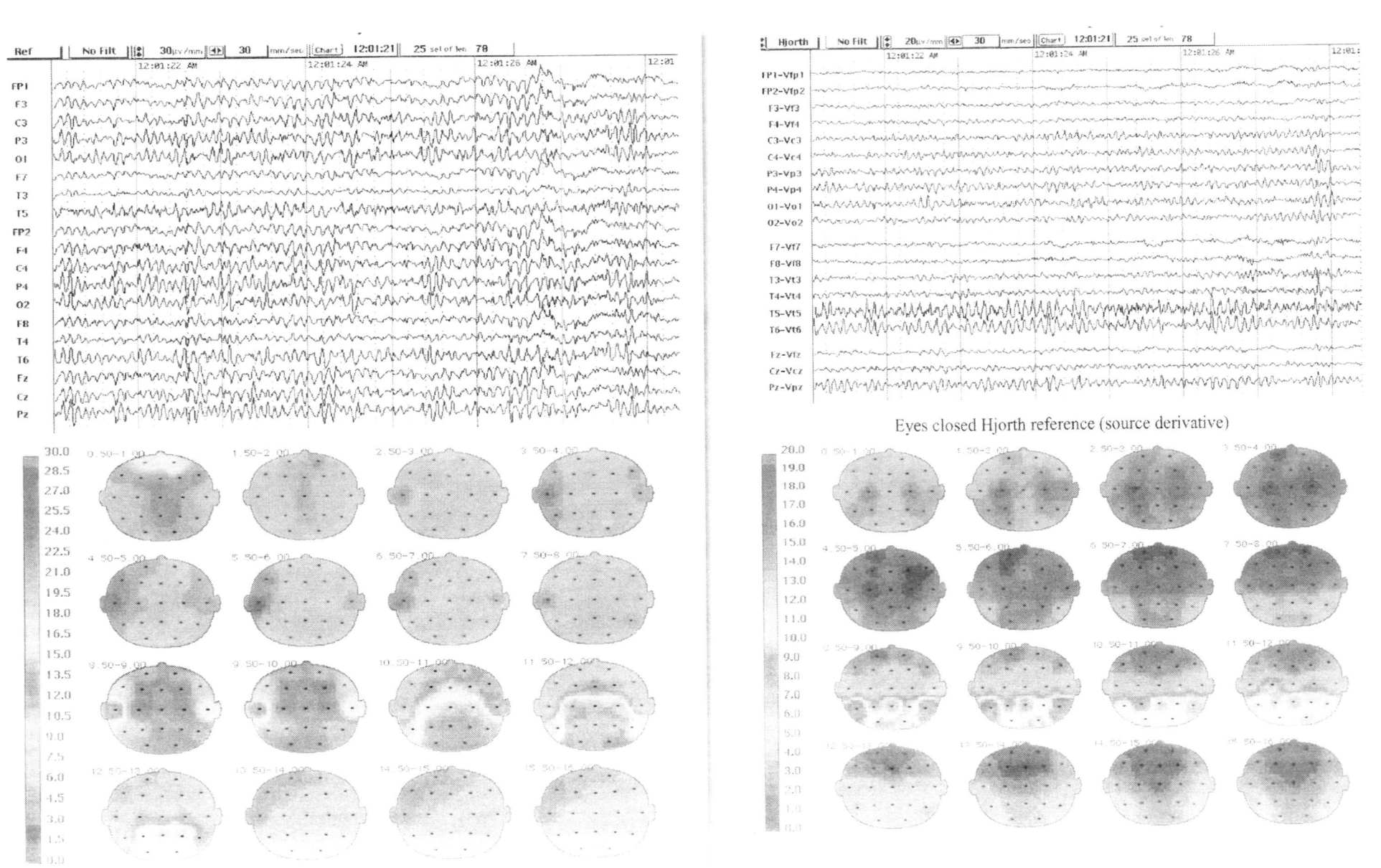

Eyes closed Hjorth reference (source derivative)

Practicum in Artifacting

In the pages that follow, printed with the Neurorep-system, you will find epochs of raw EEG data that have been selected from several different patients. They are in a referential montage, and the EO line at the bottom is a bipolar eye movement channel. Please note that no page numbers will appear and that the record number is in the upper right corner. We want you to take one record at a time, study each epoch and identify first, whether the epoch contains artifacts and should be rejected, or if it should be accepted. Second, determine for yourself on scratch paper what types of artifact are present in each rejected epoch. After artifacting each page, turn to the end of the section and compare your findings with ours. We will tell you which epochs we accepted on each page and identify the artifacts present. In many cases we have also guided you to which channels to examine to see the artifacts. Continue in this manner, artifacting one page at a time, and then comparing your results with ours until you have completed the exercise. The examples of raw EEG were printed using the NeuroRep program of Bill Hudspeth, PhD.

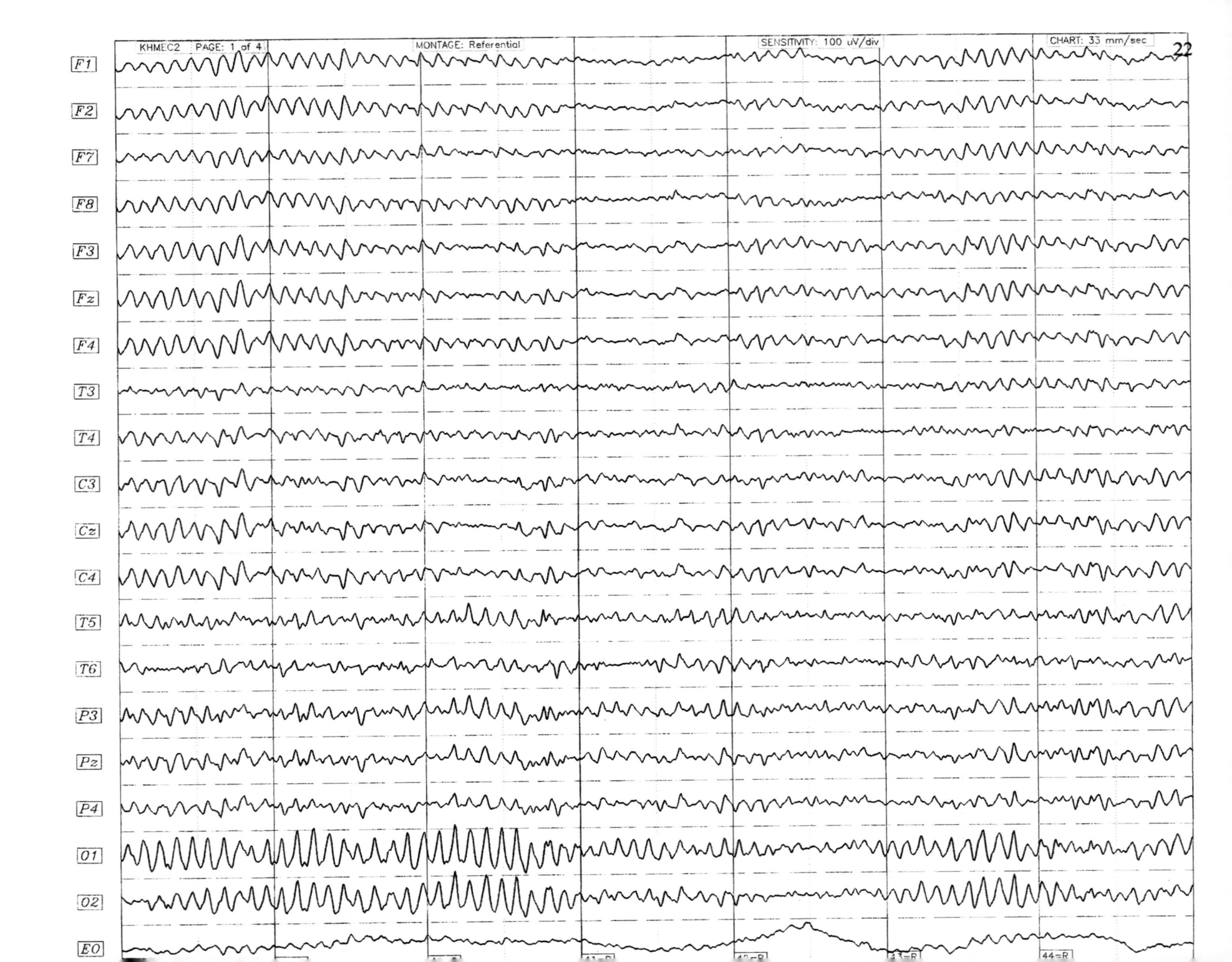

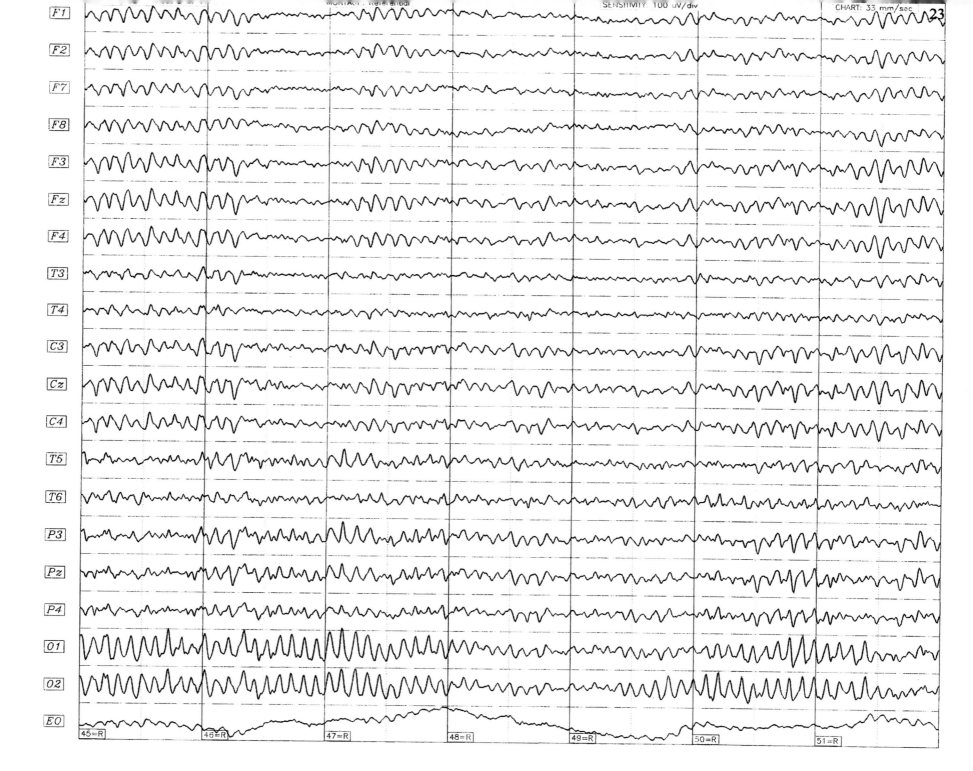

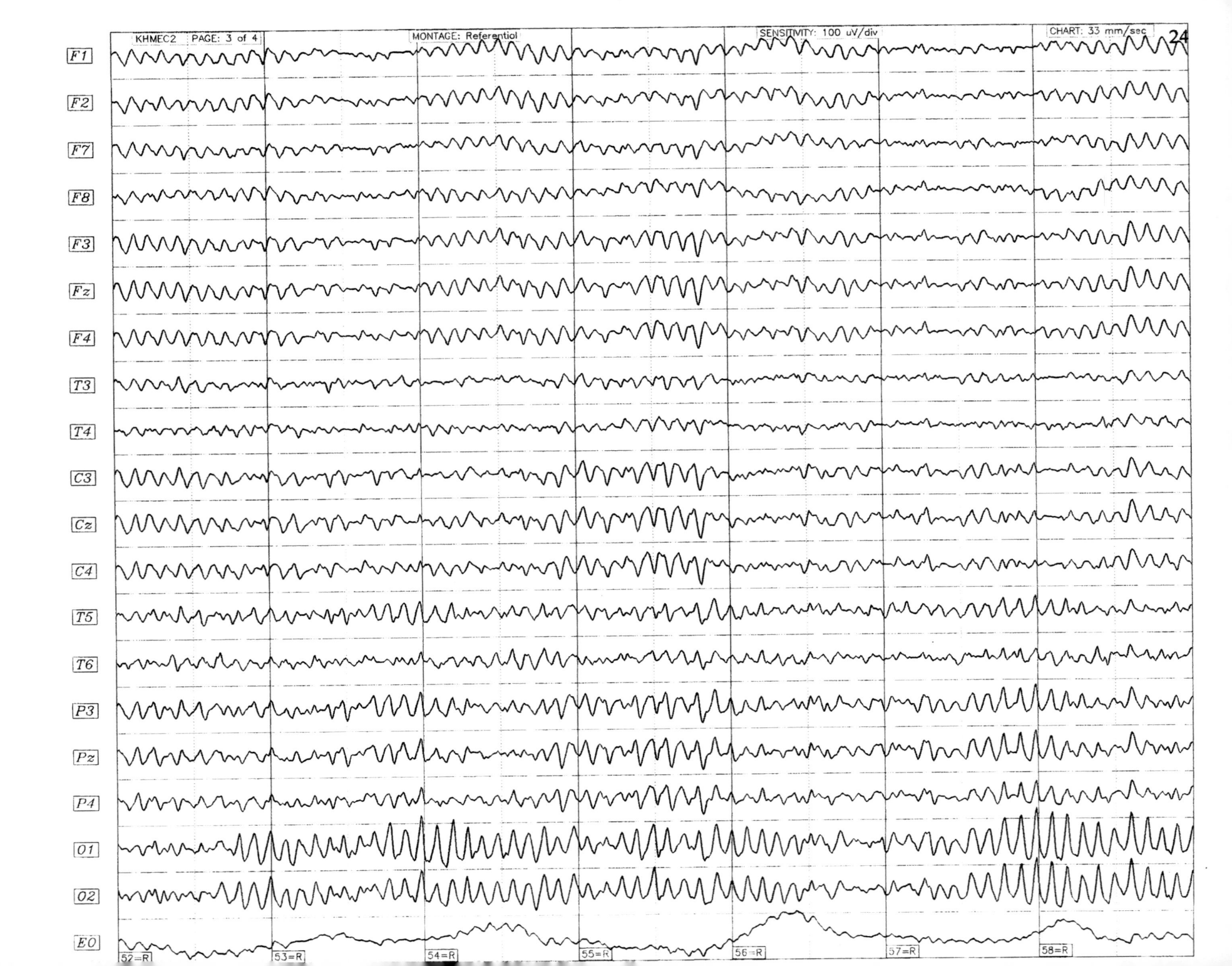

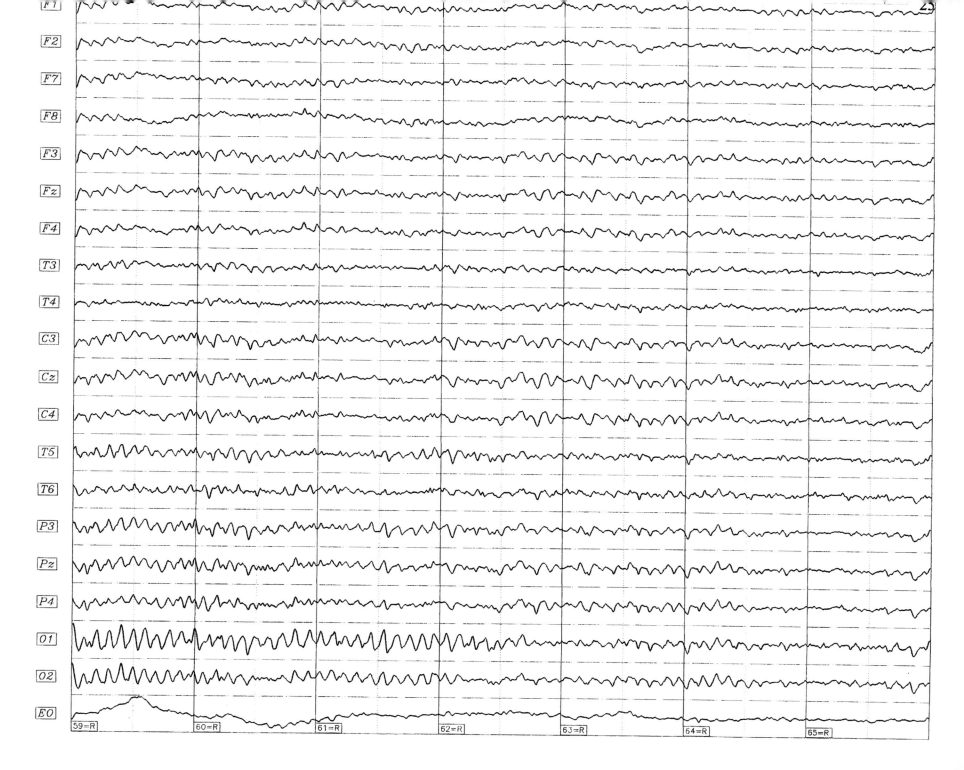

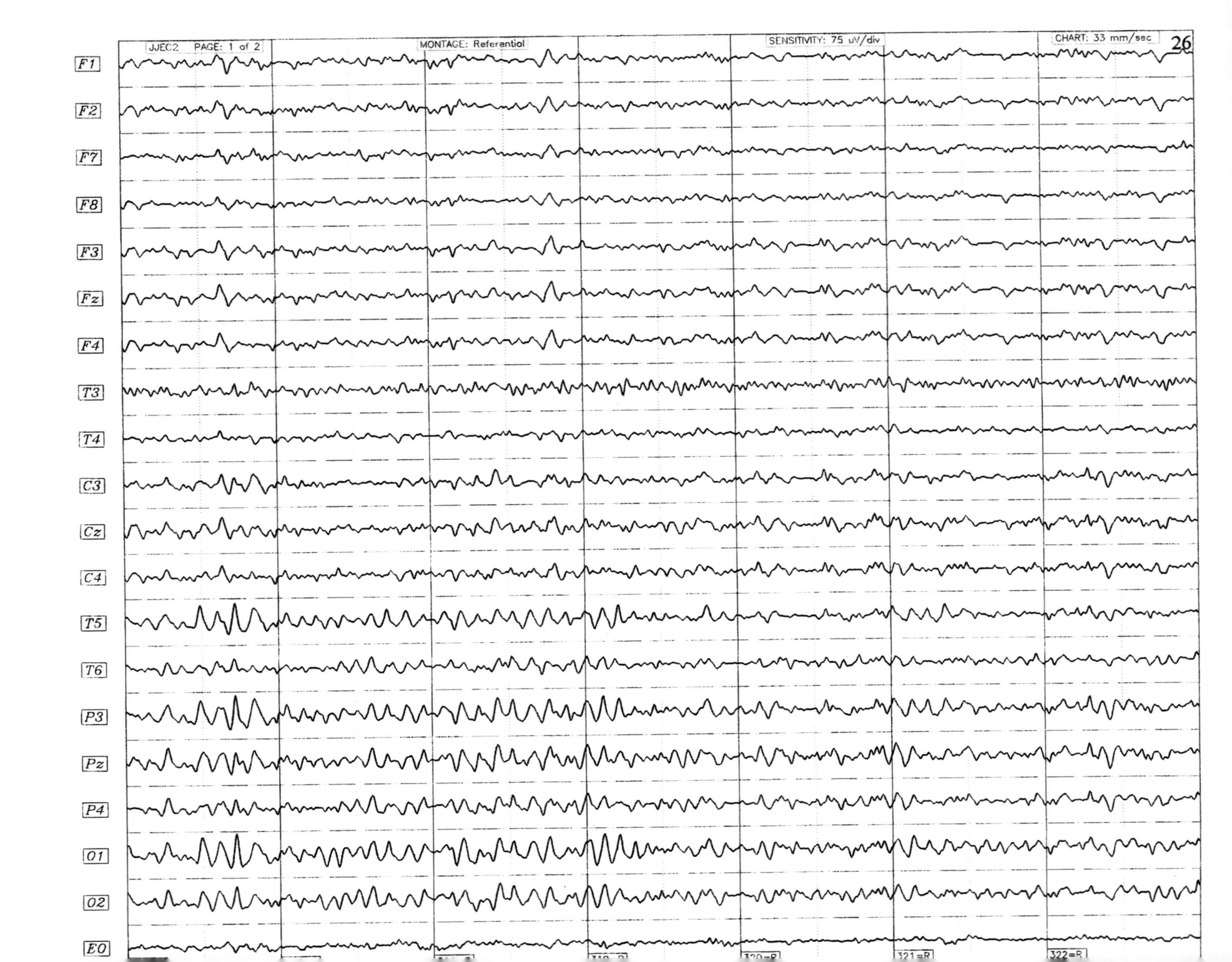

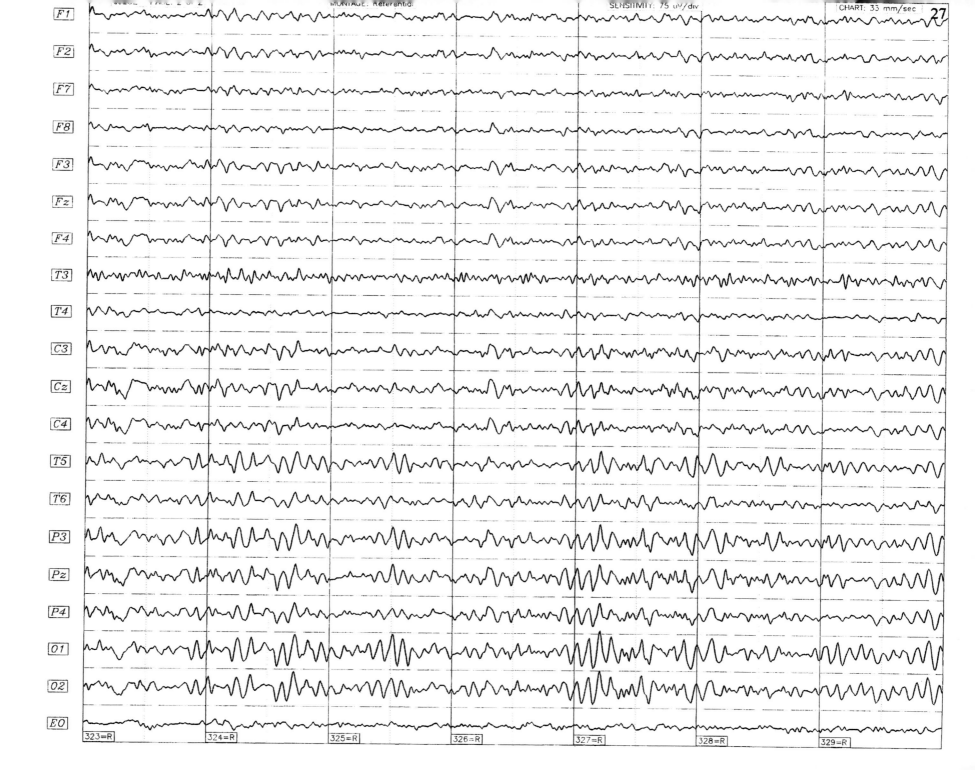

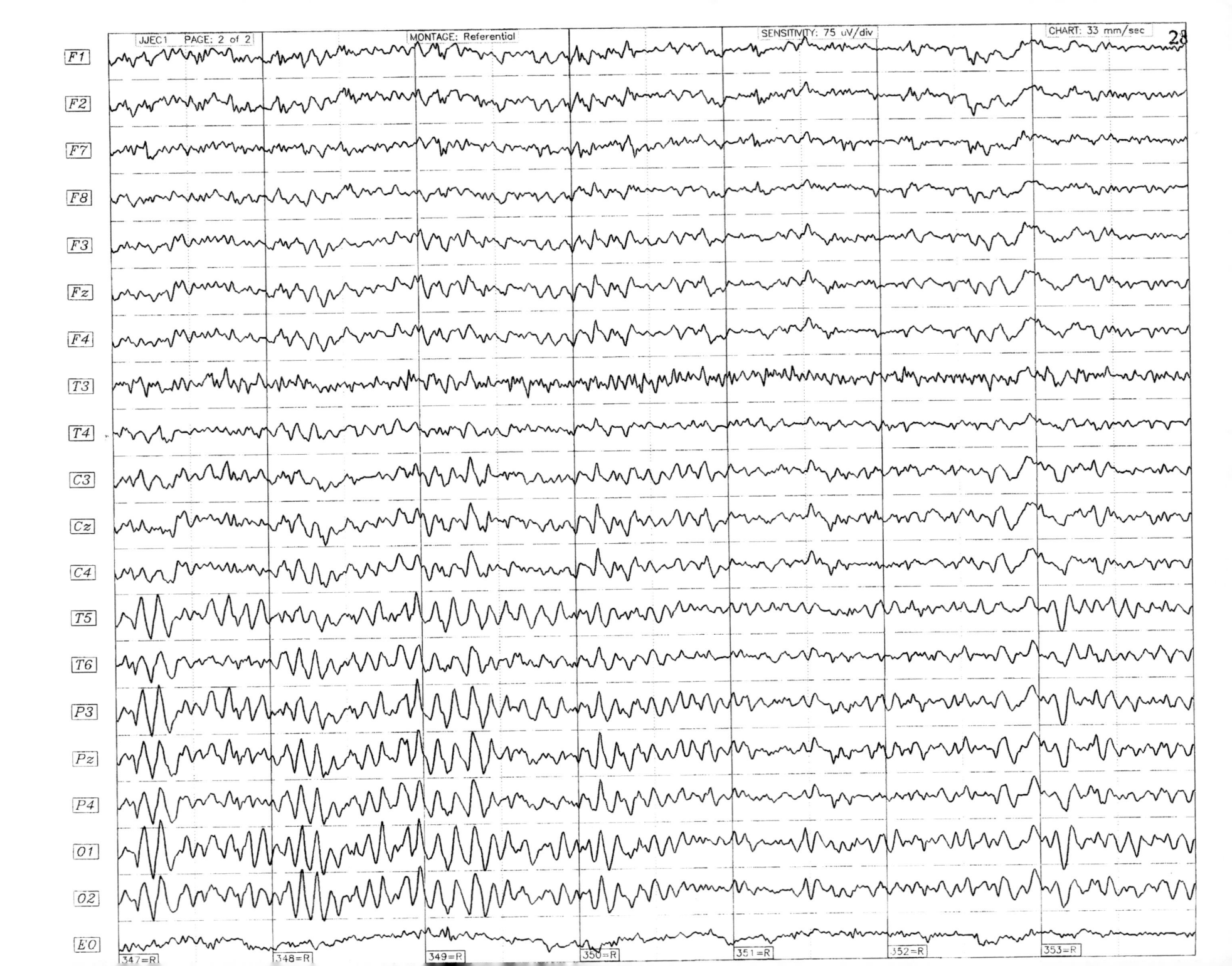

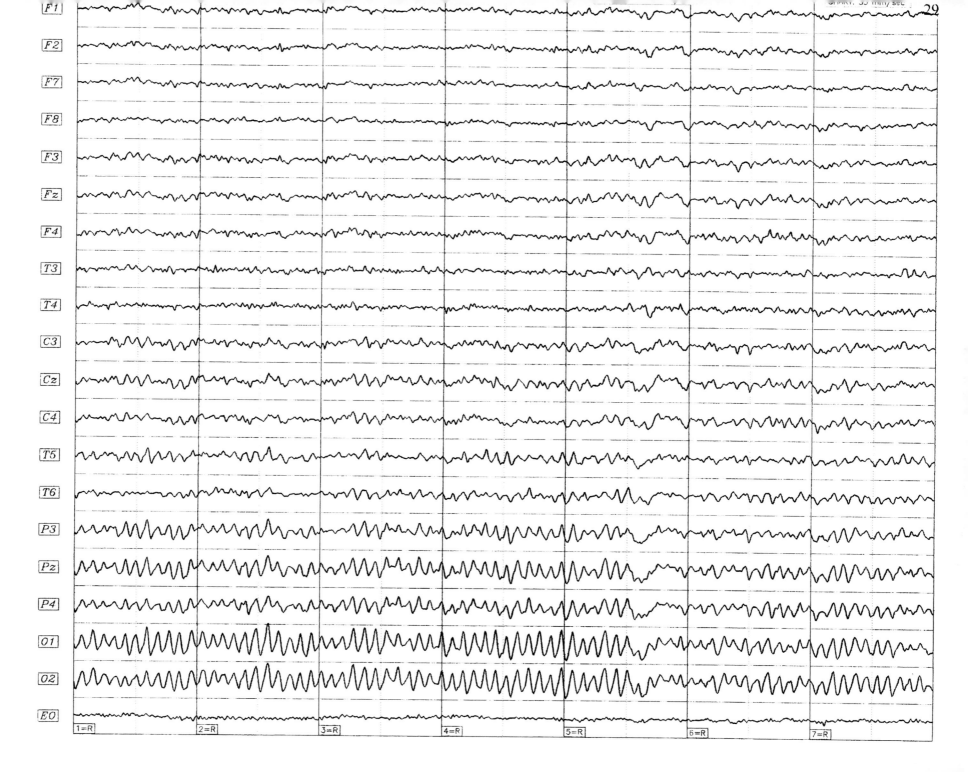

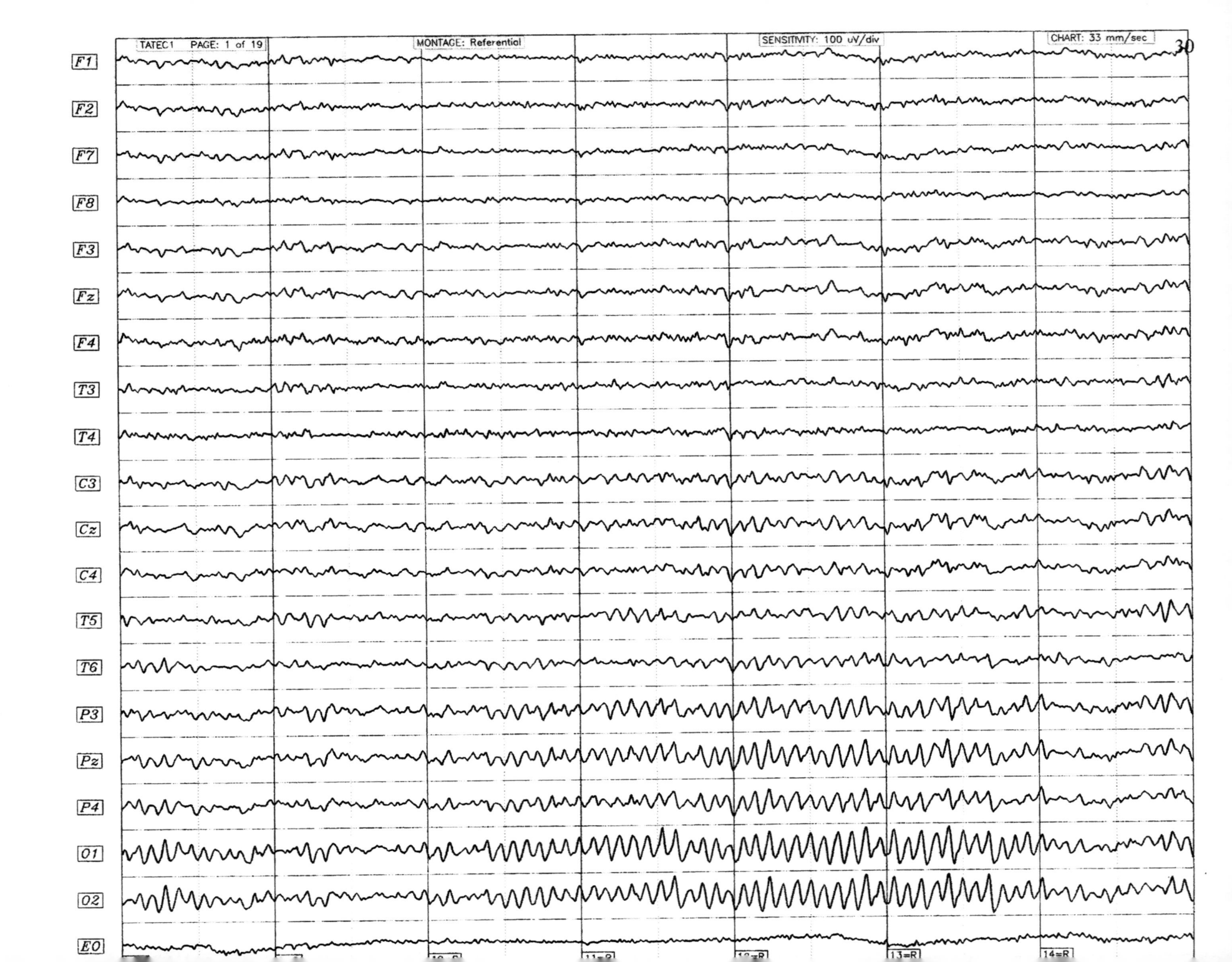

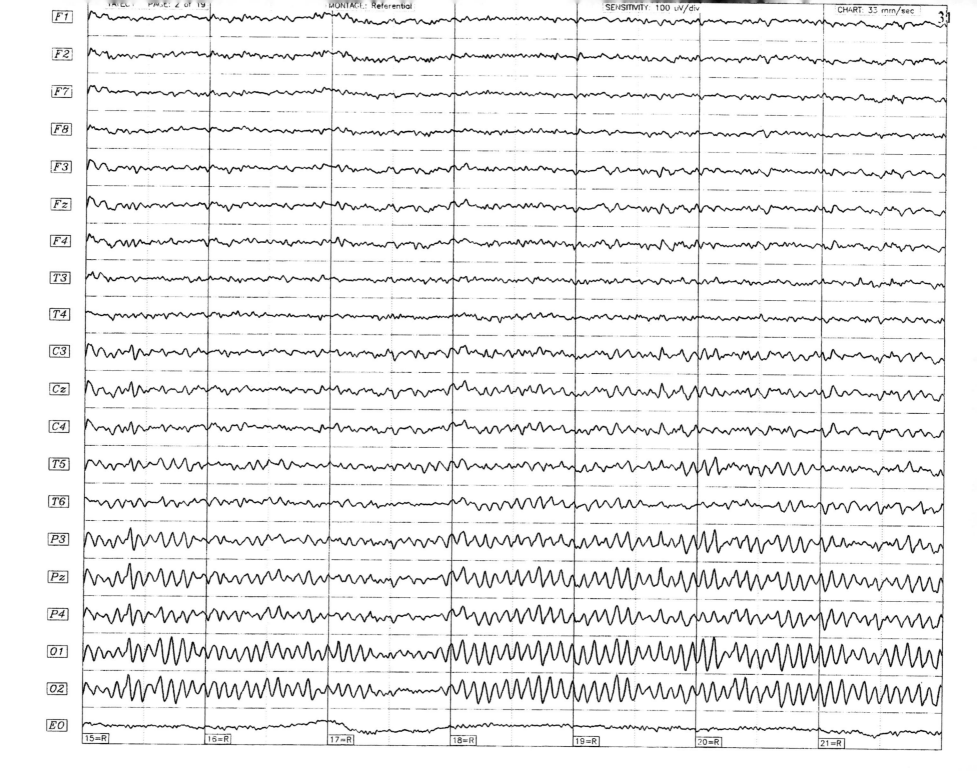

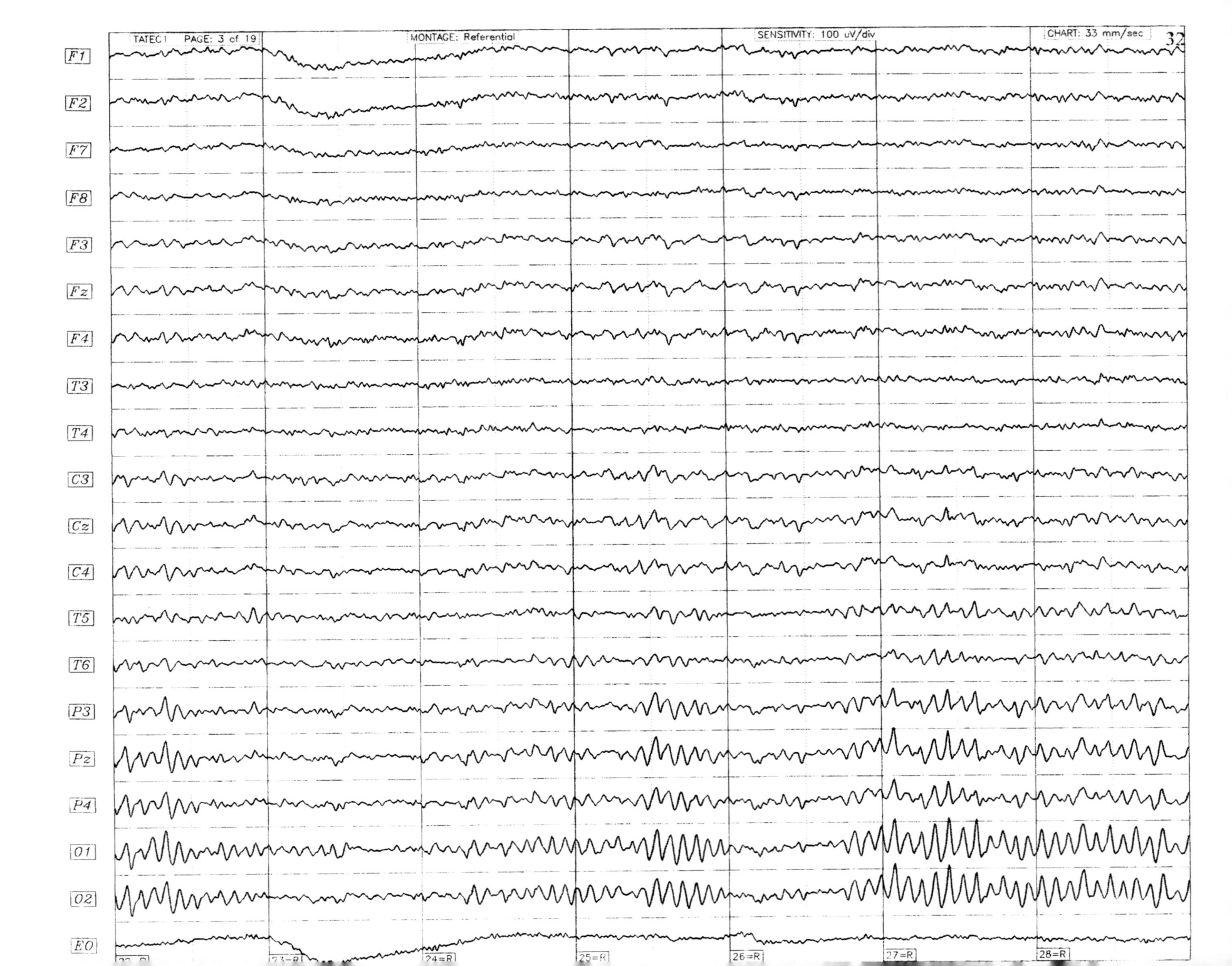

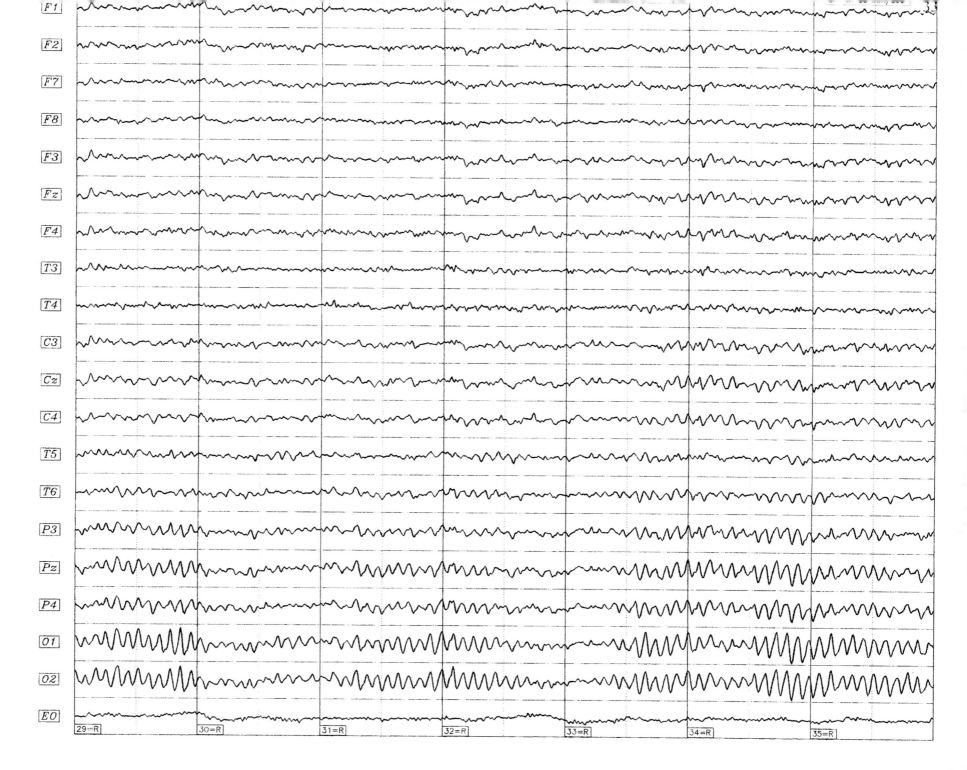

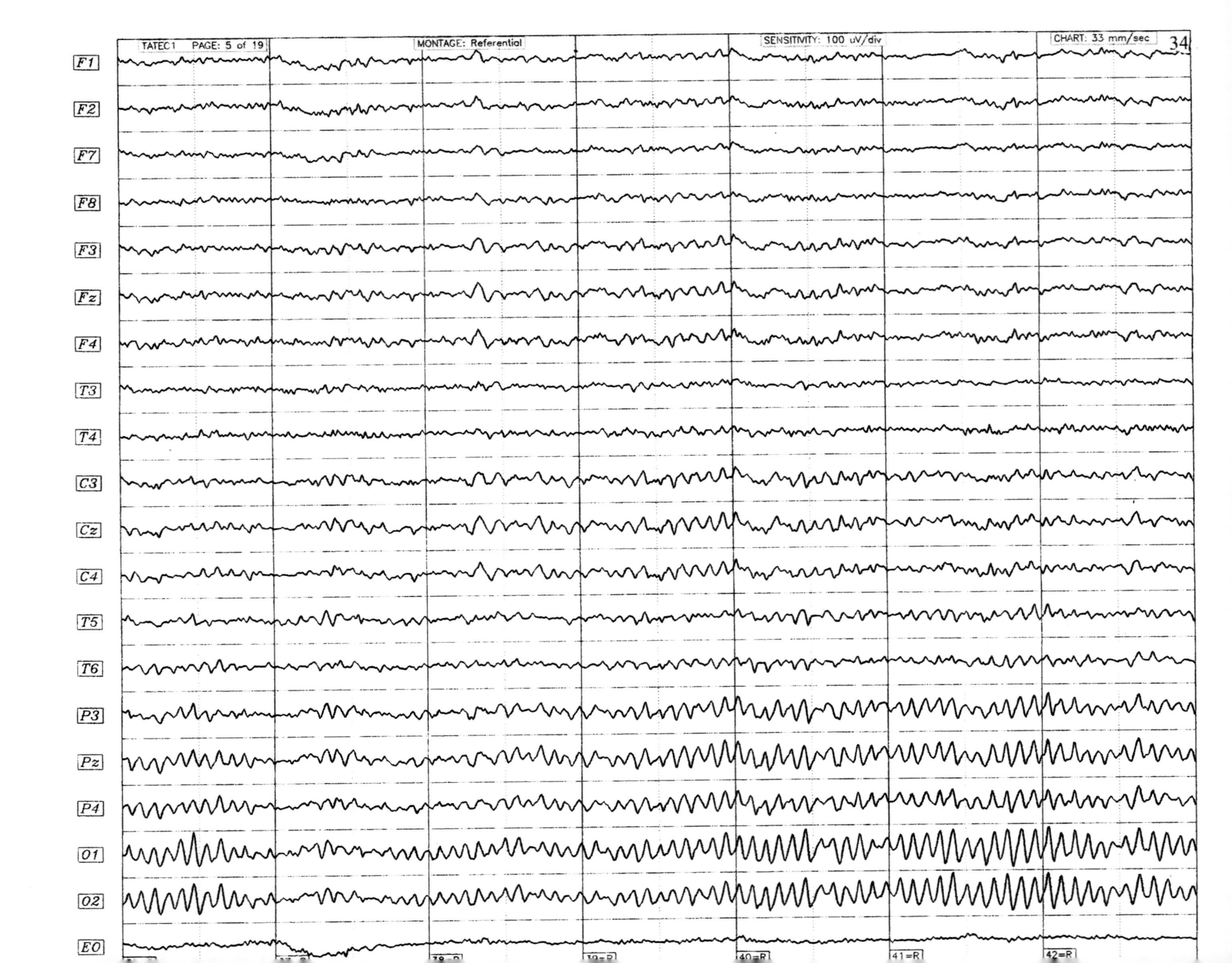

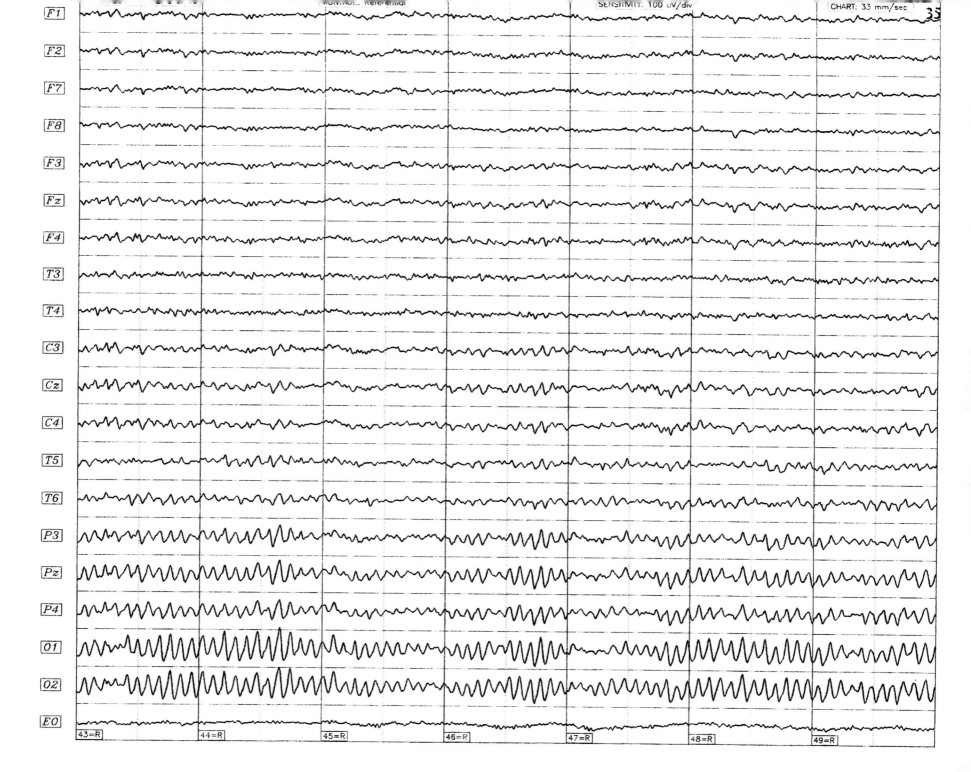

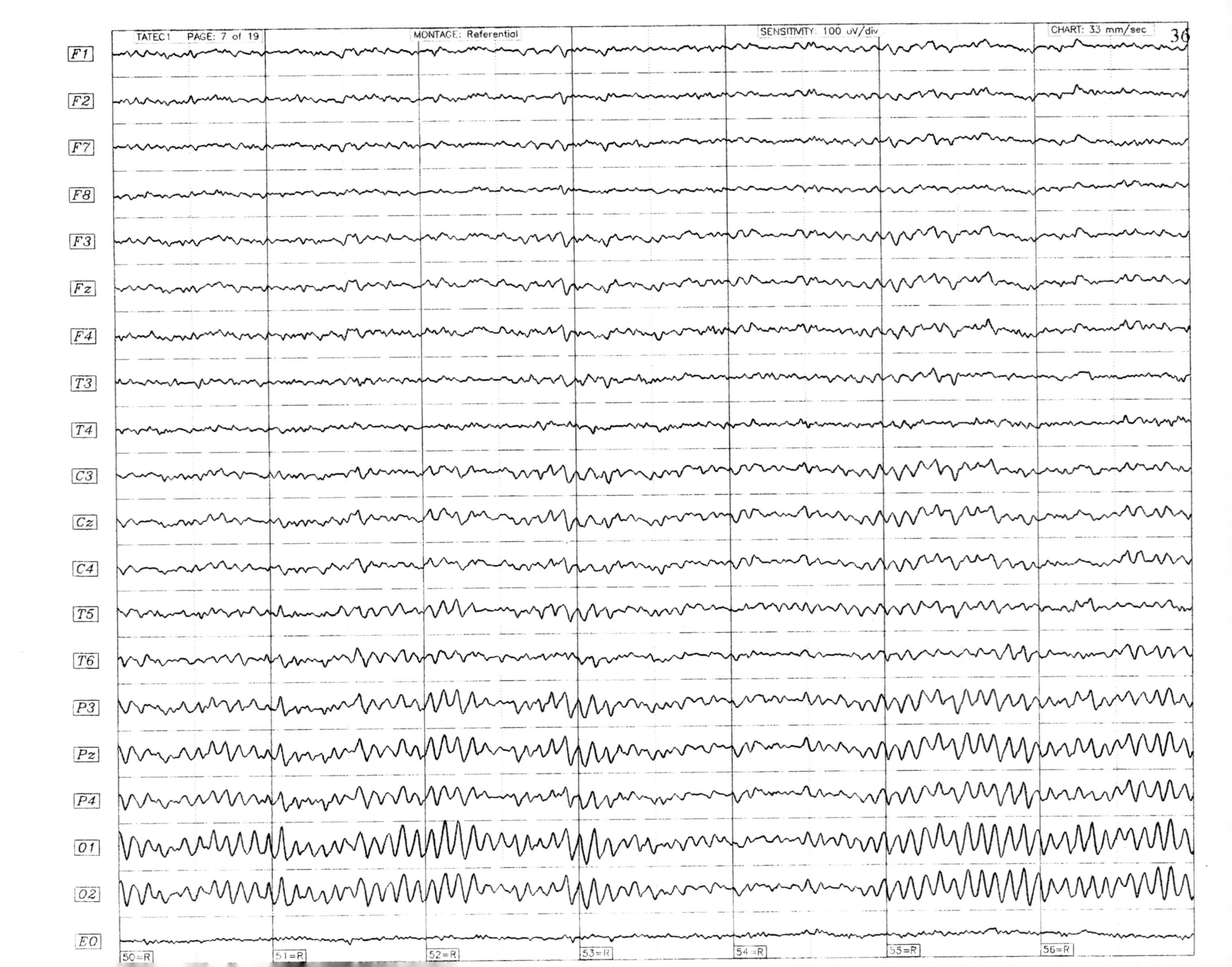

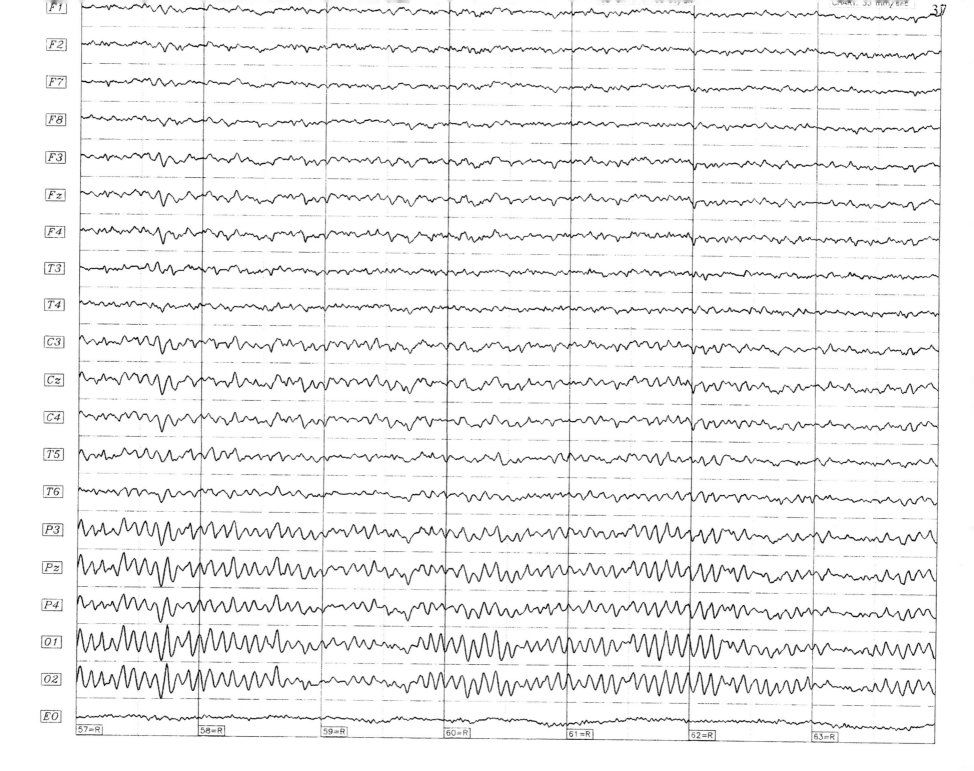

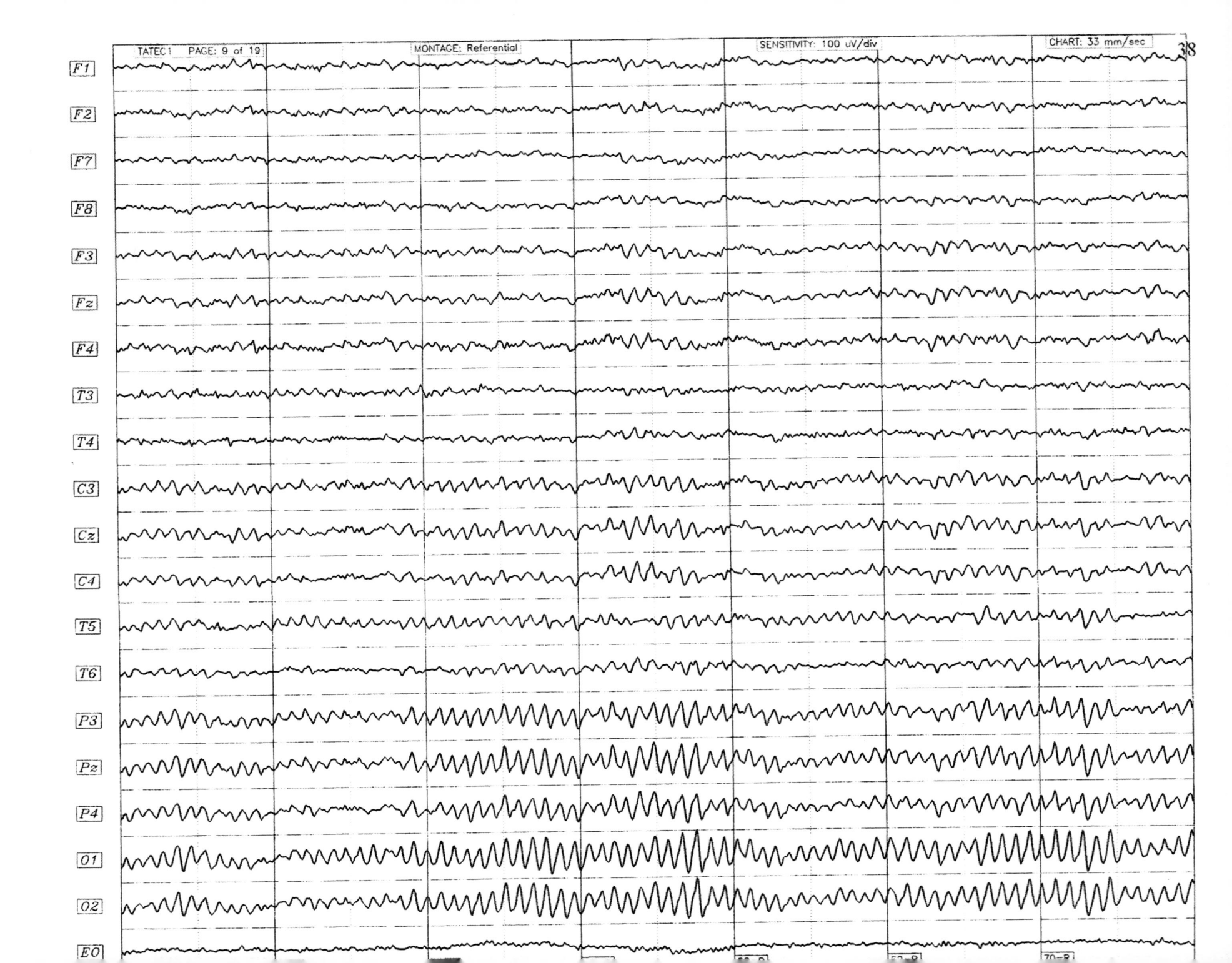

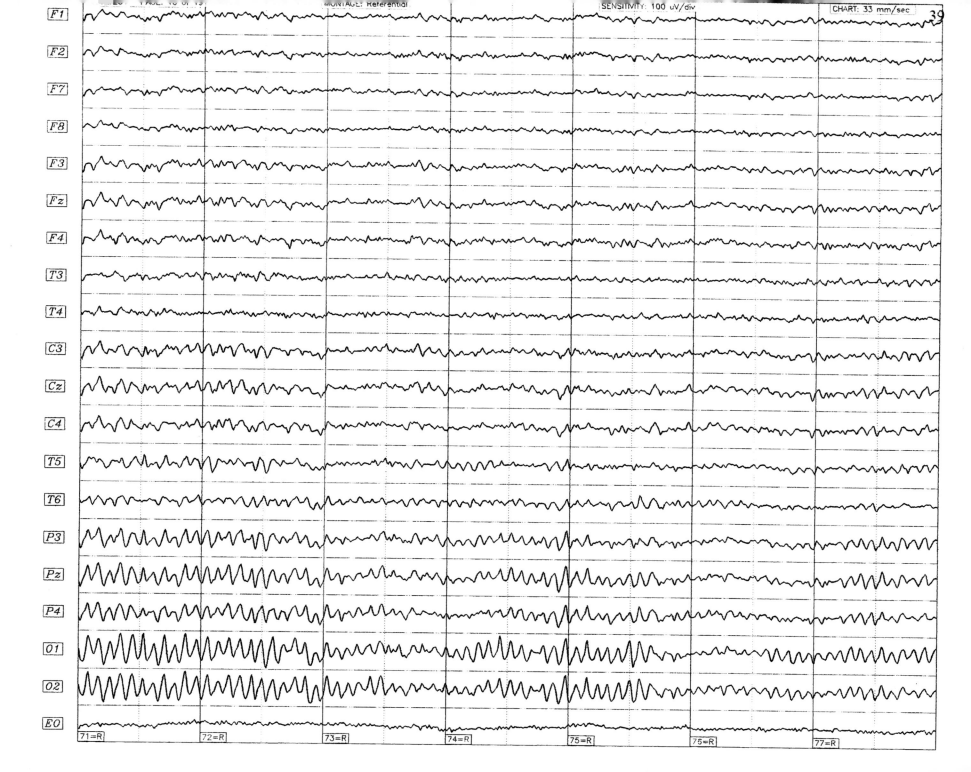

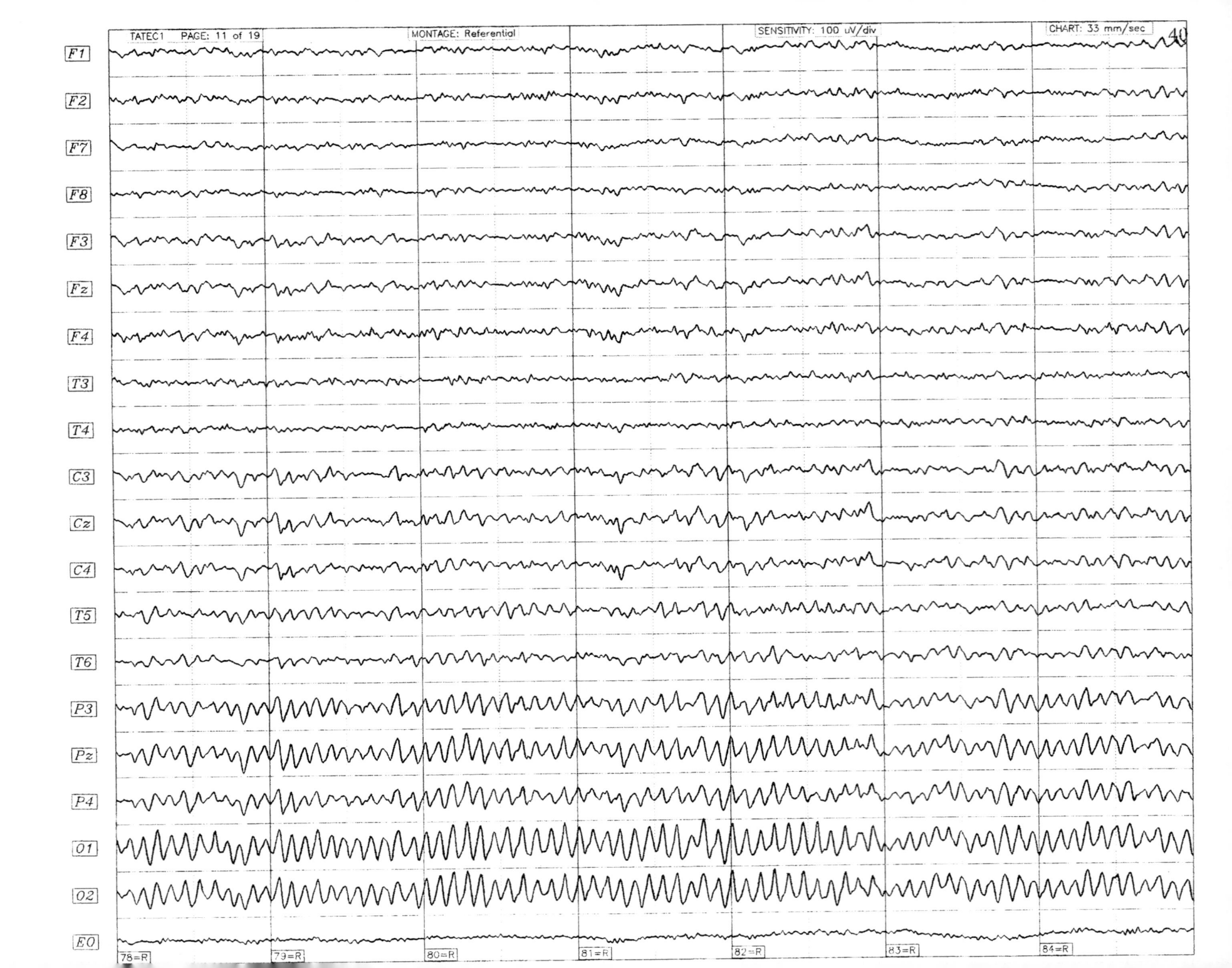

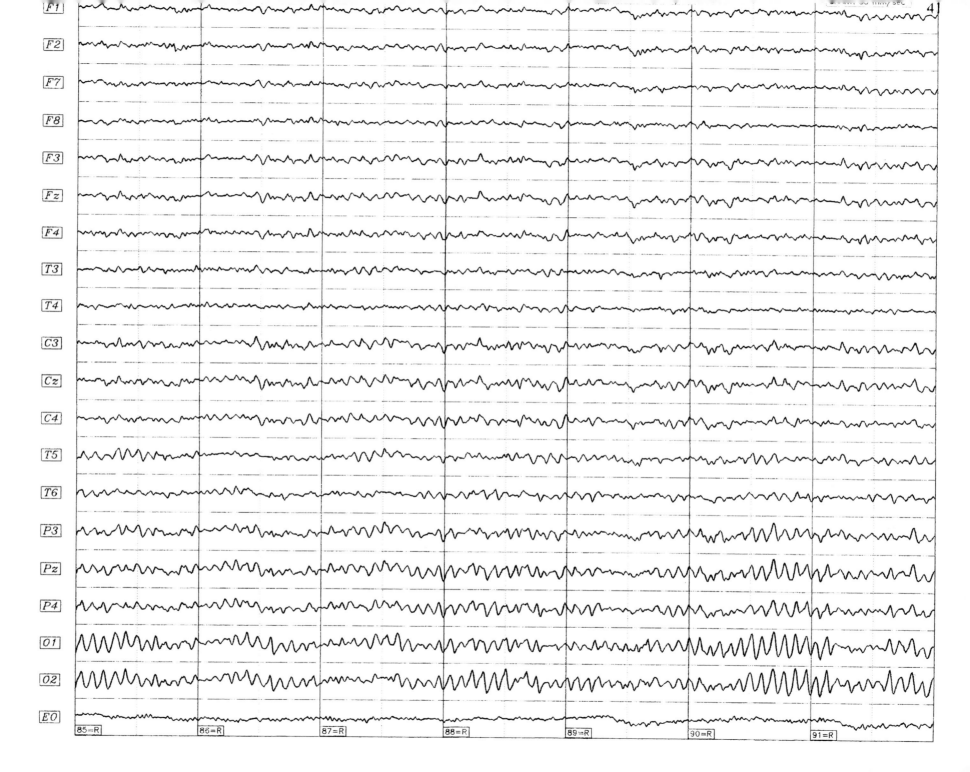

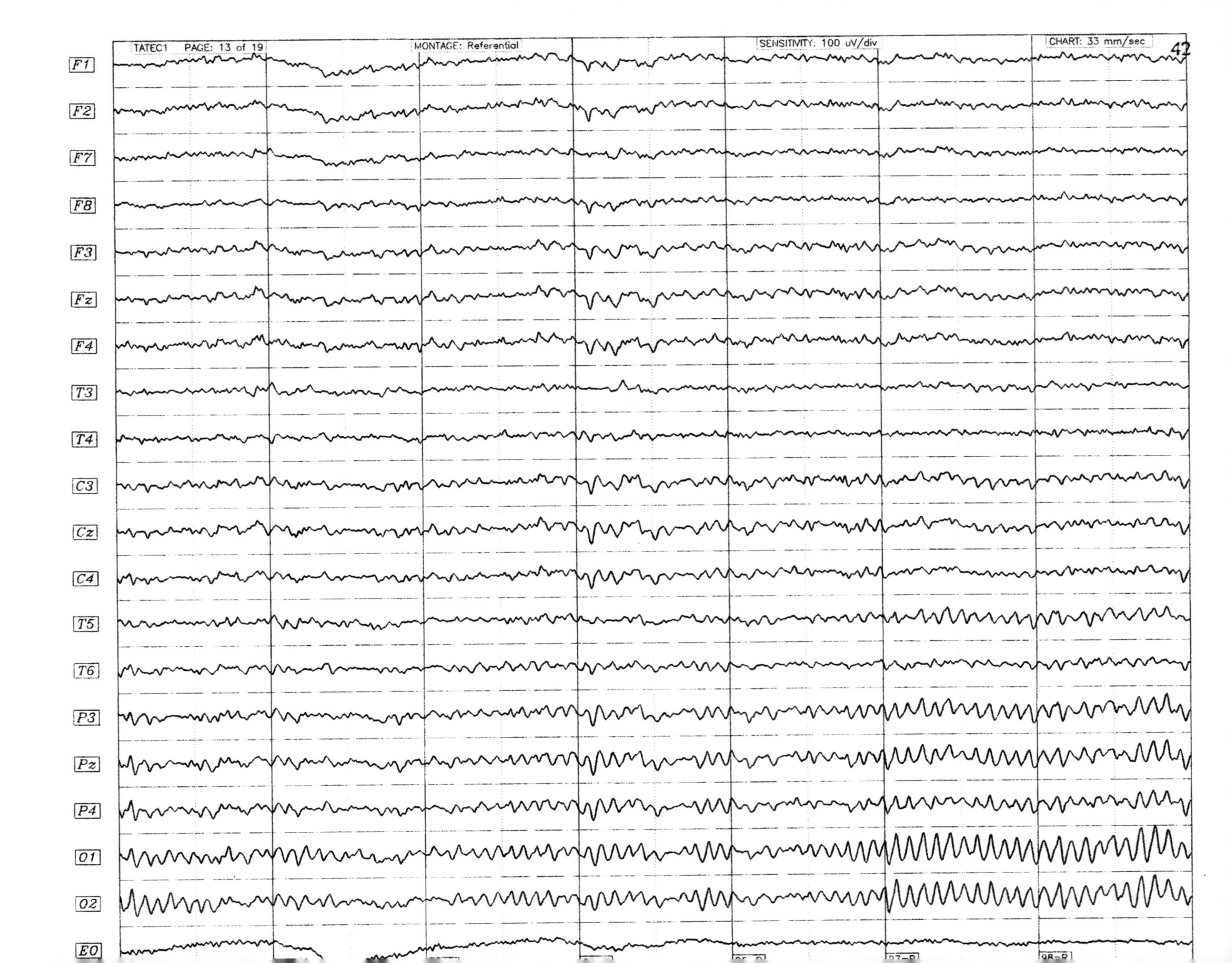

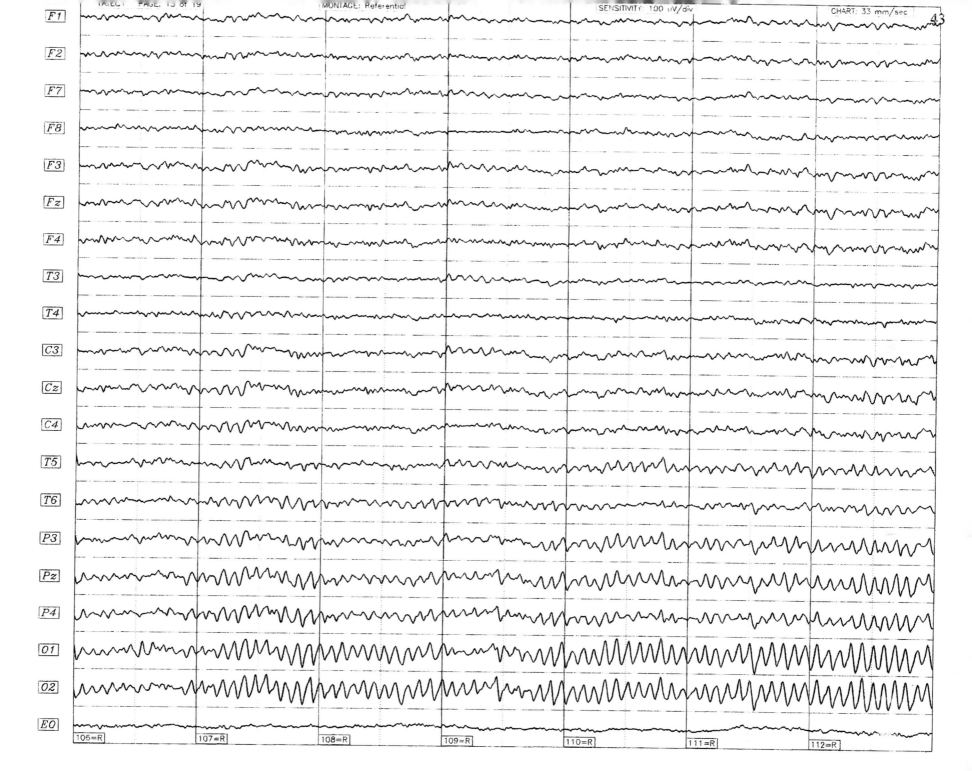

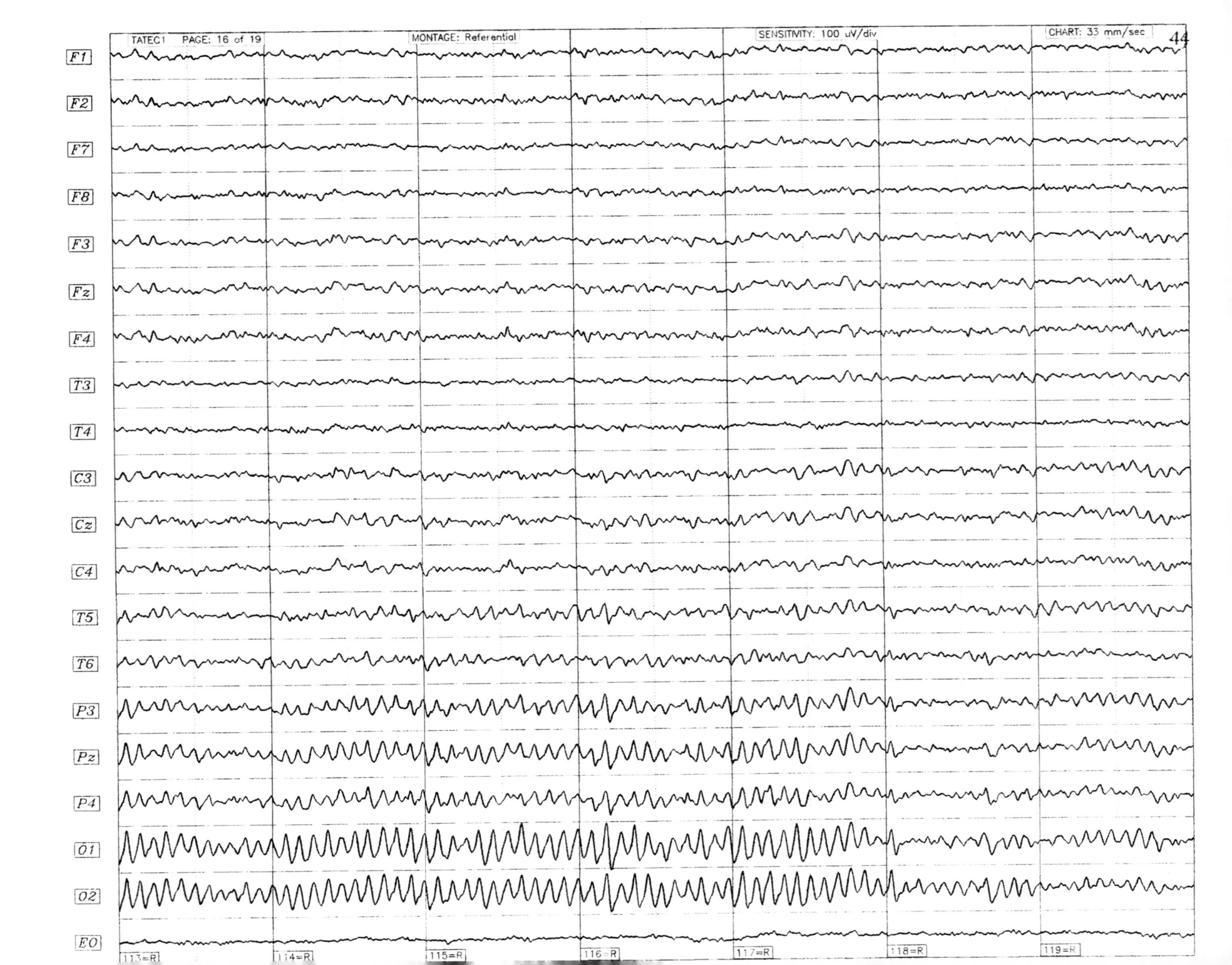

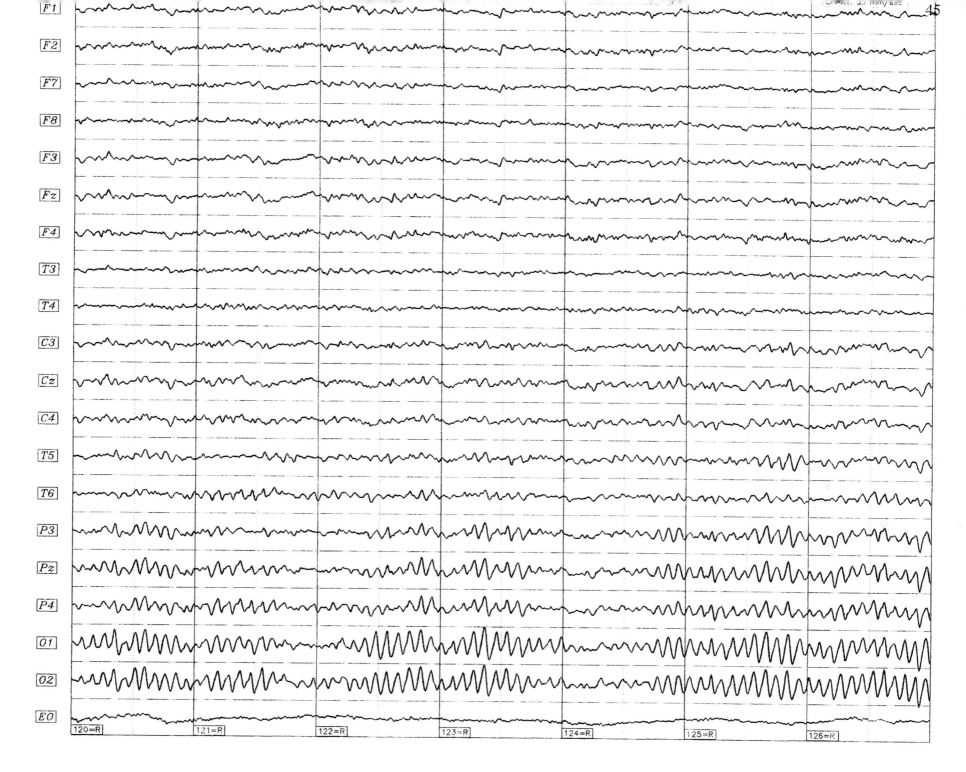

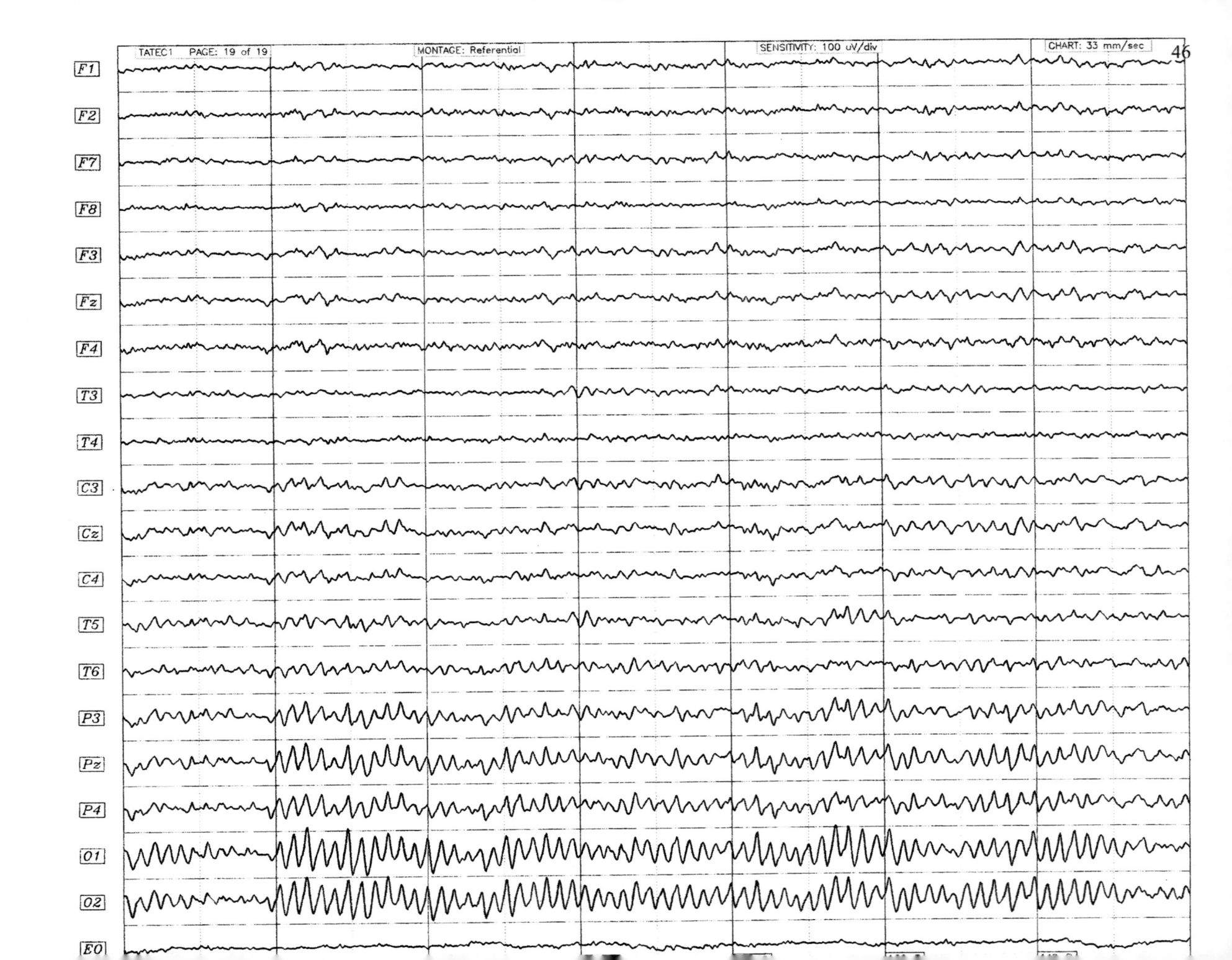

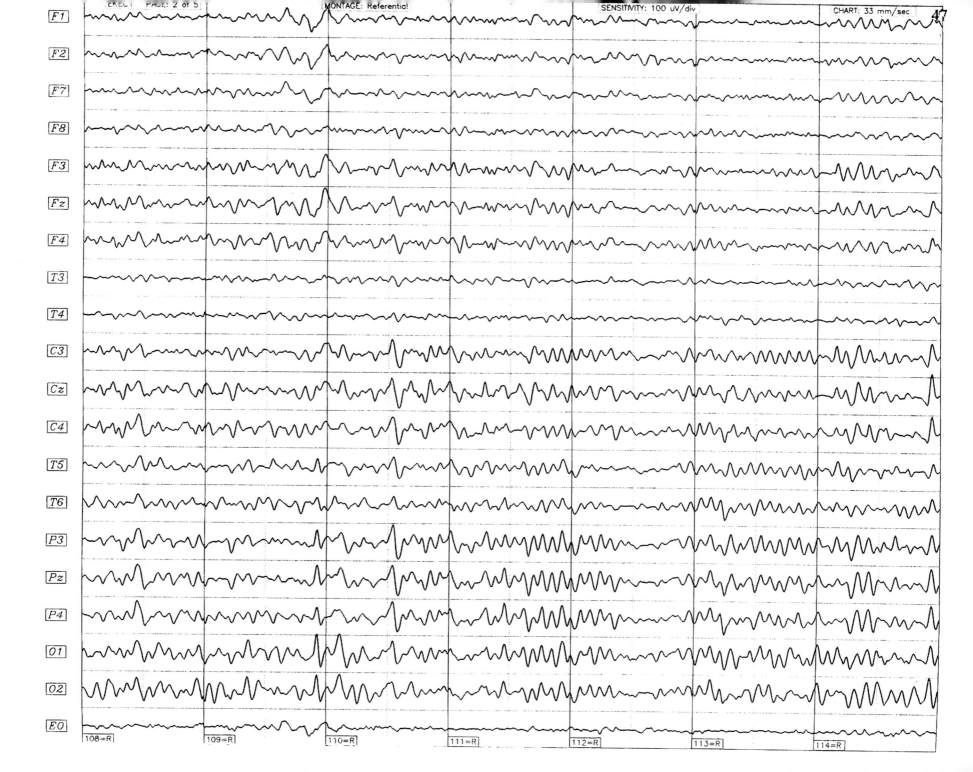

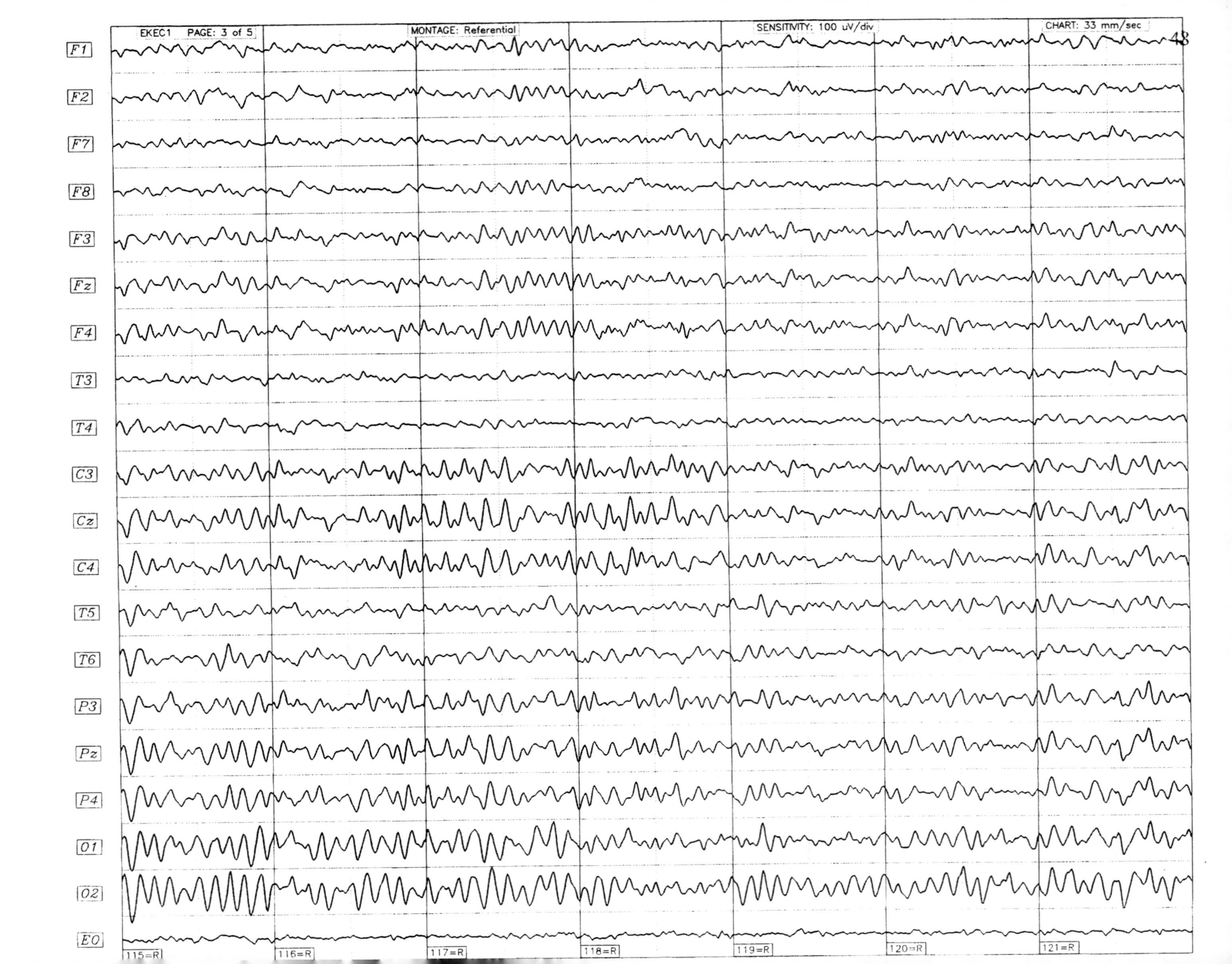

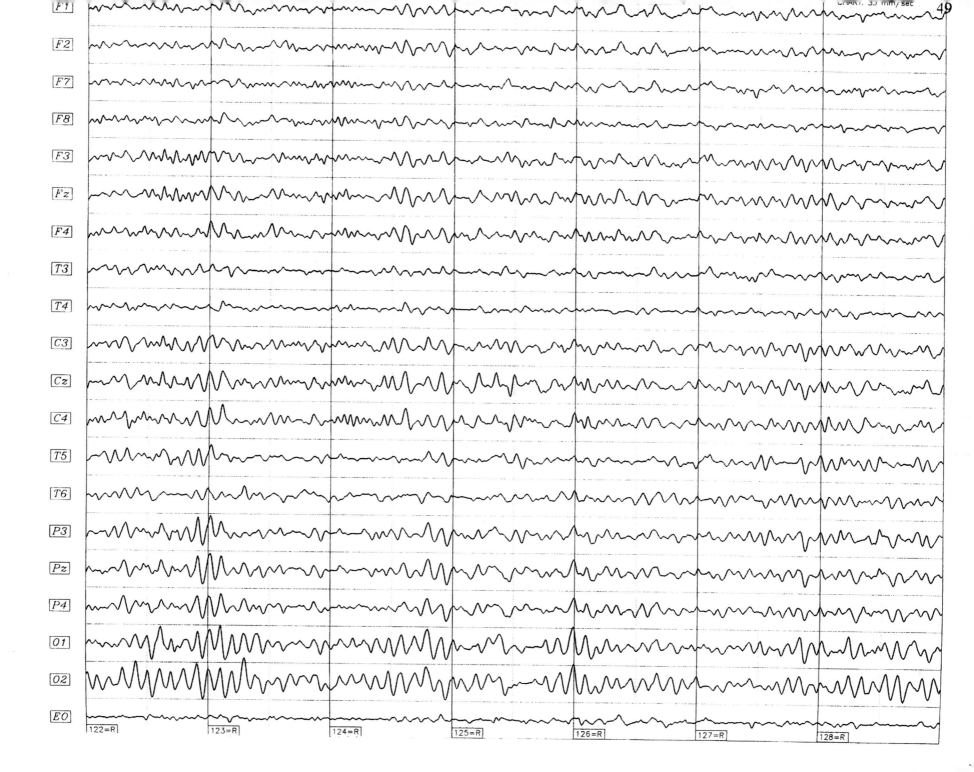

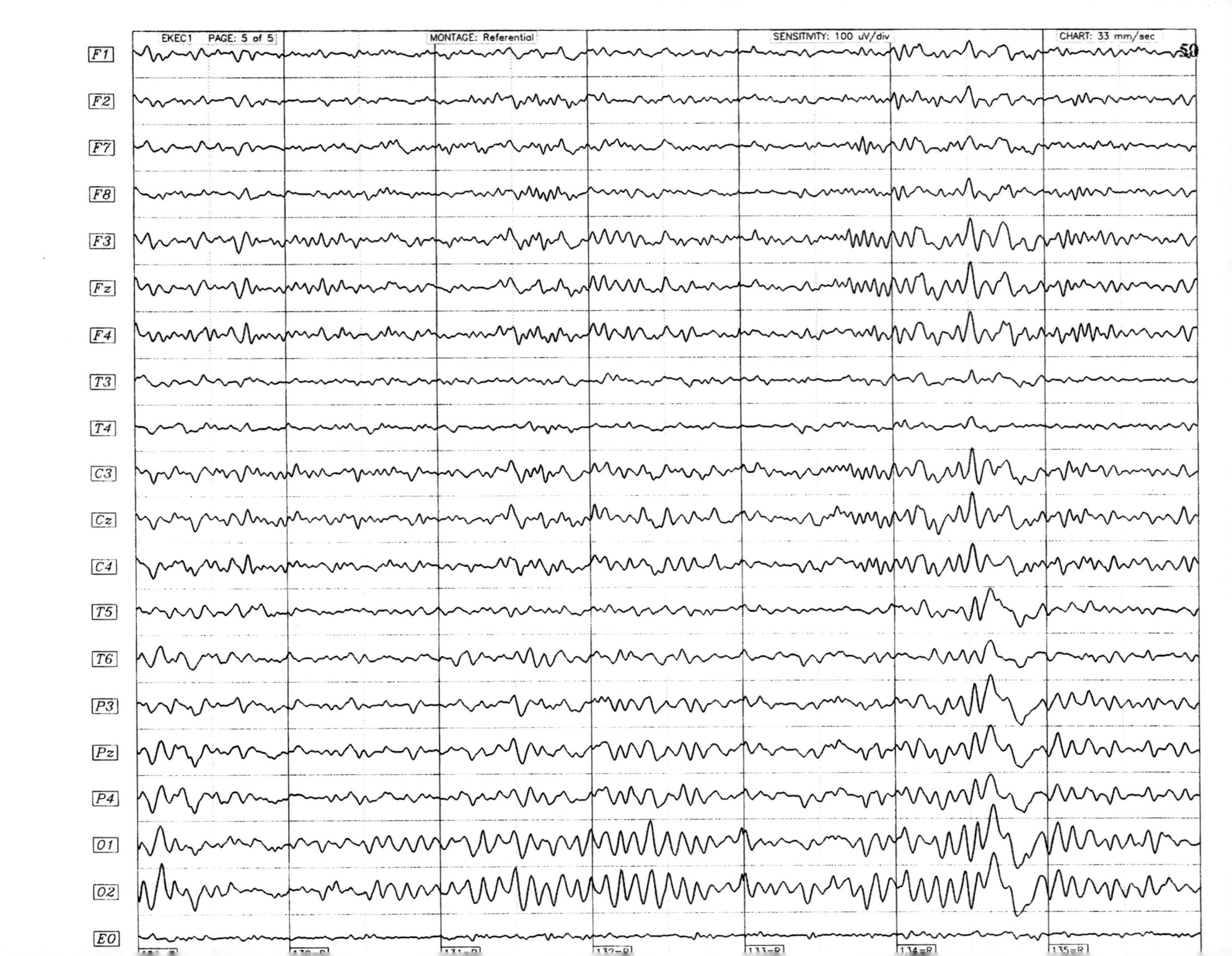

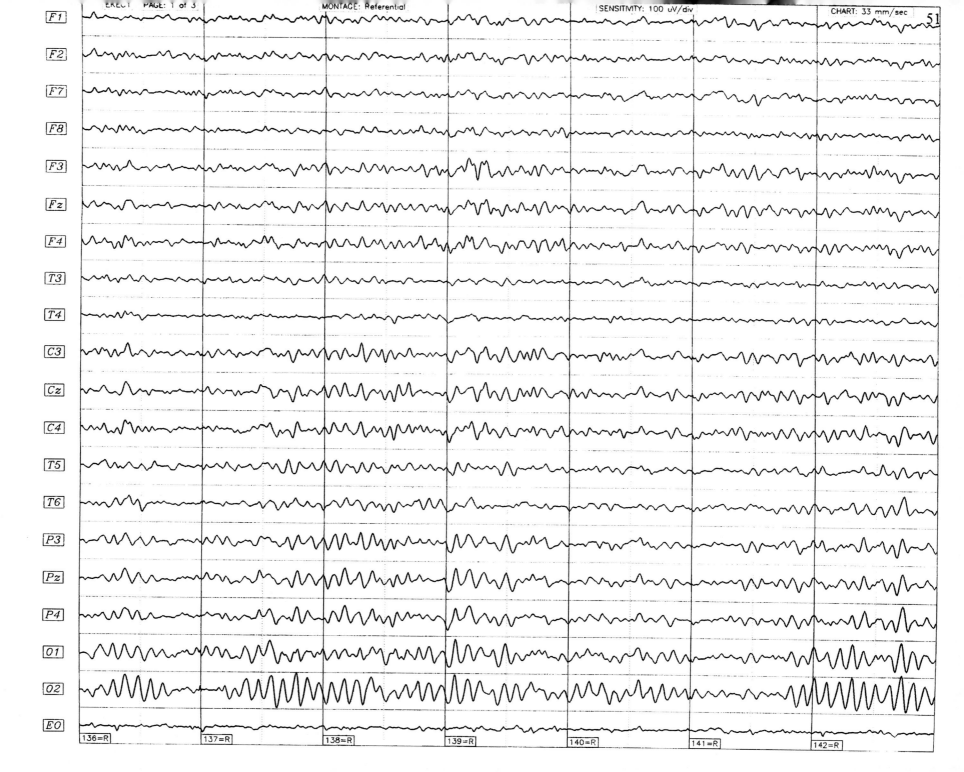

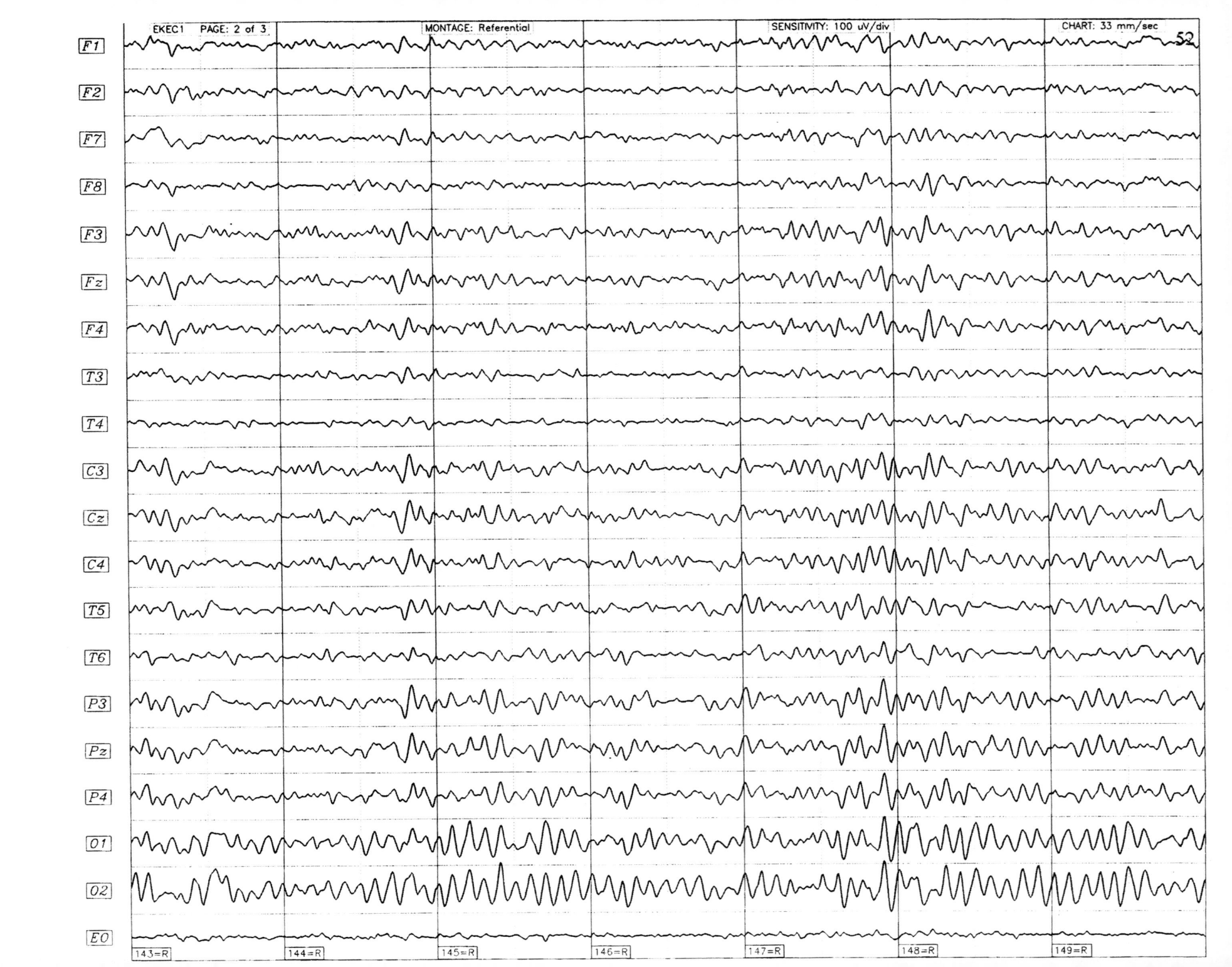

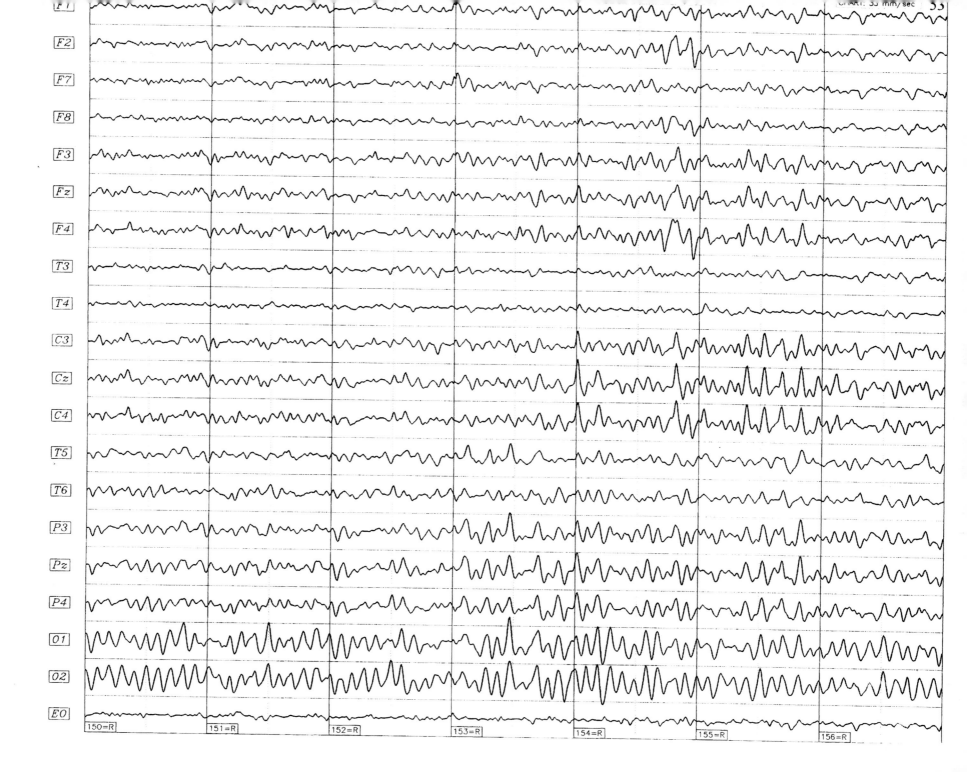

F1
F2
F7
F8
F3
Fz
F4
T3
T4
C3
Cz
C4
T5
T6
P3
Pz
P4
O1
O2
EO

150=R   151=R   152=R   153=R   154=R   155=R   156=R

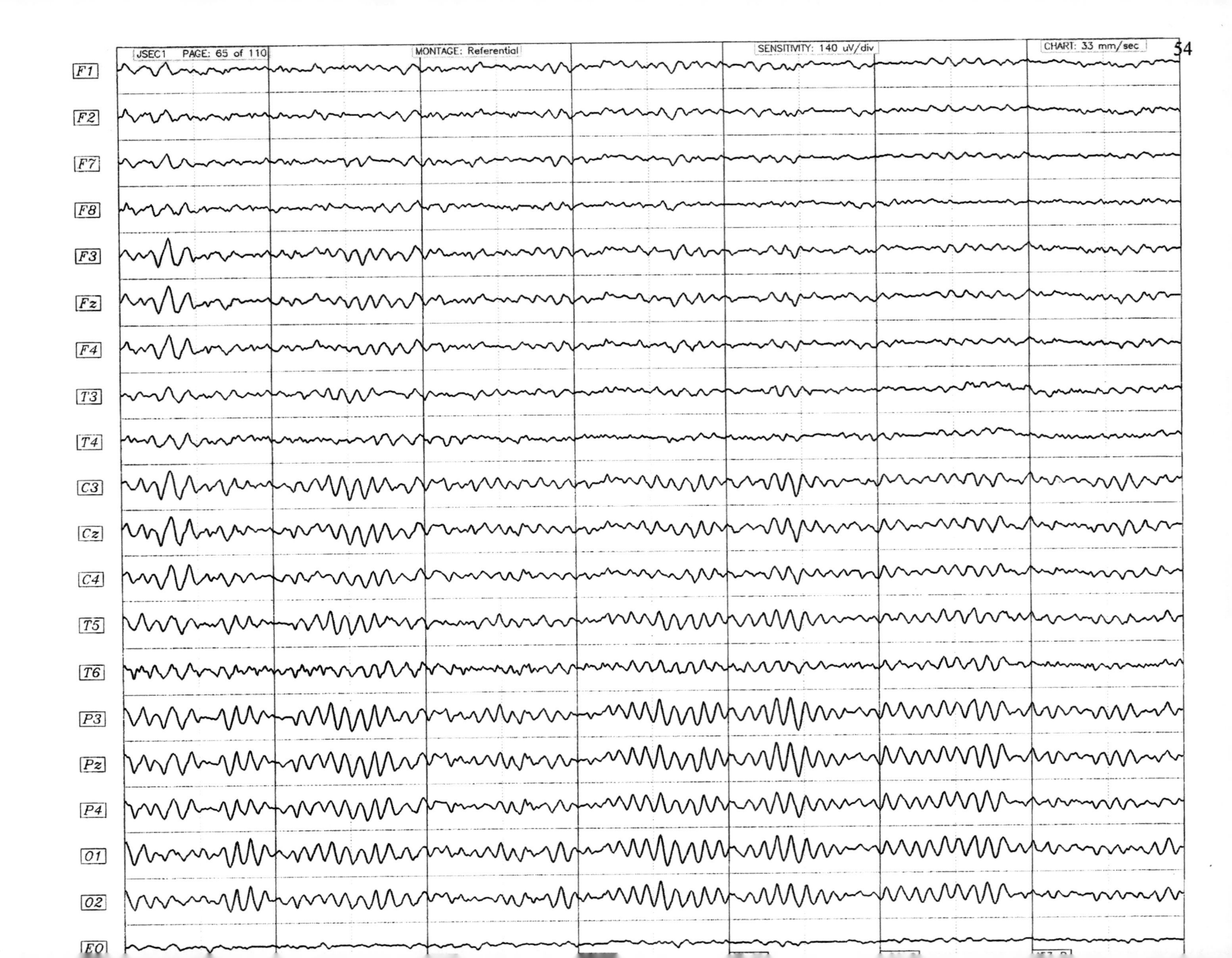

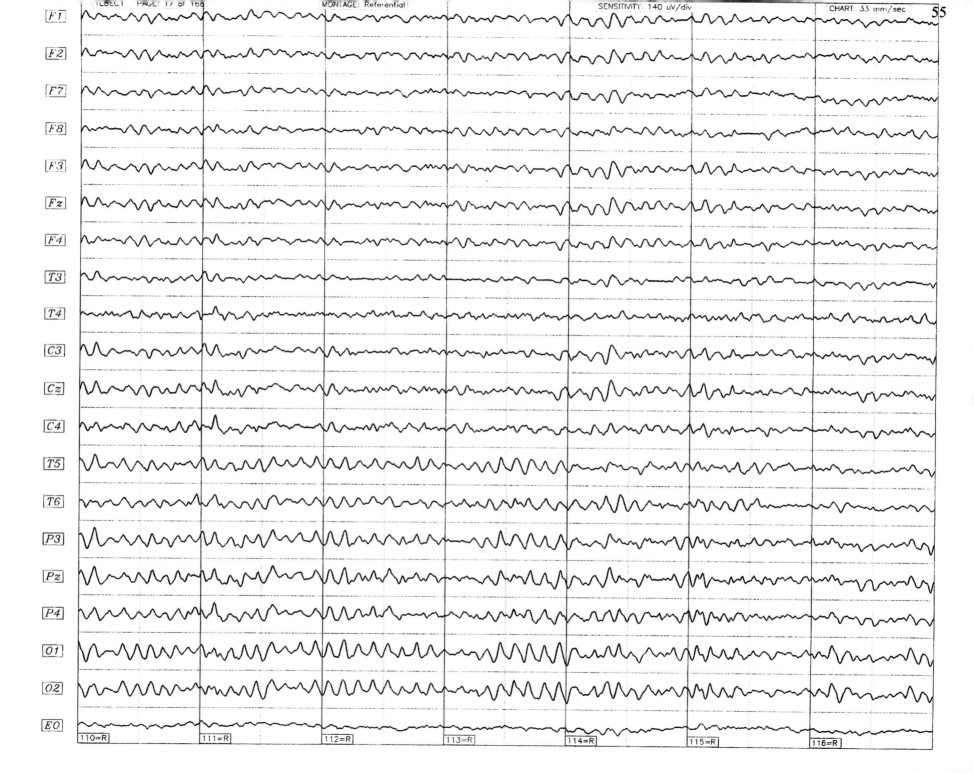

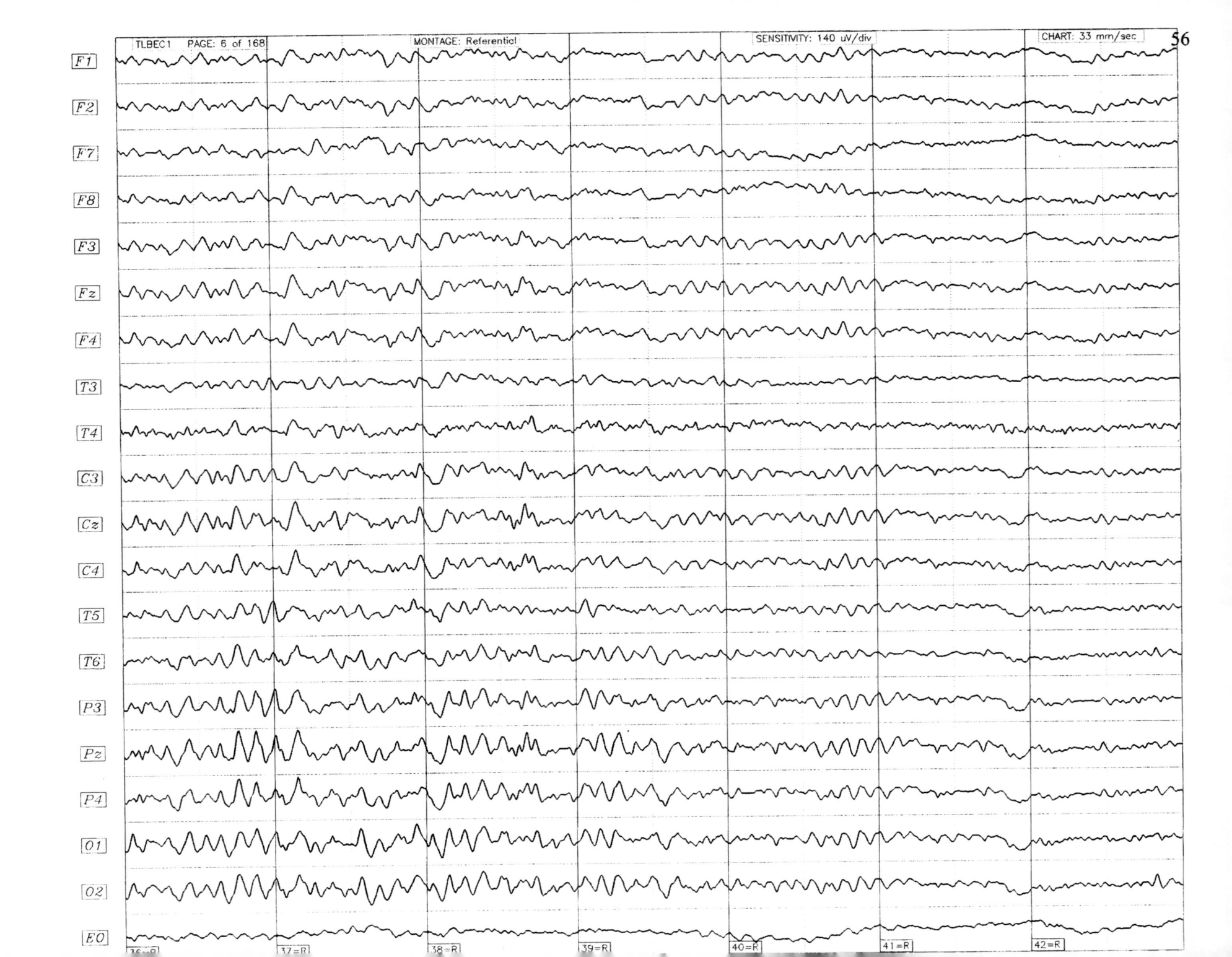

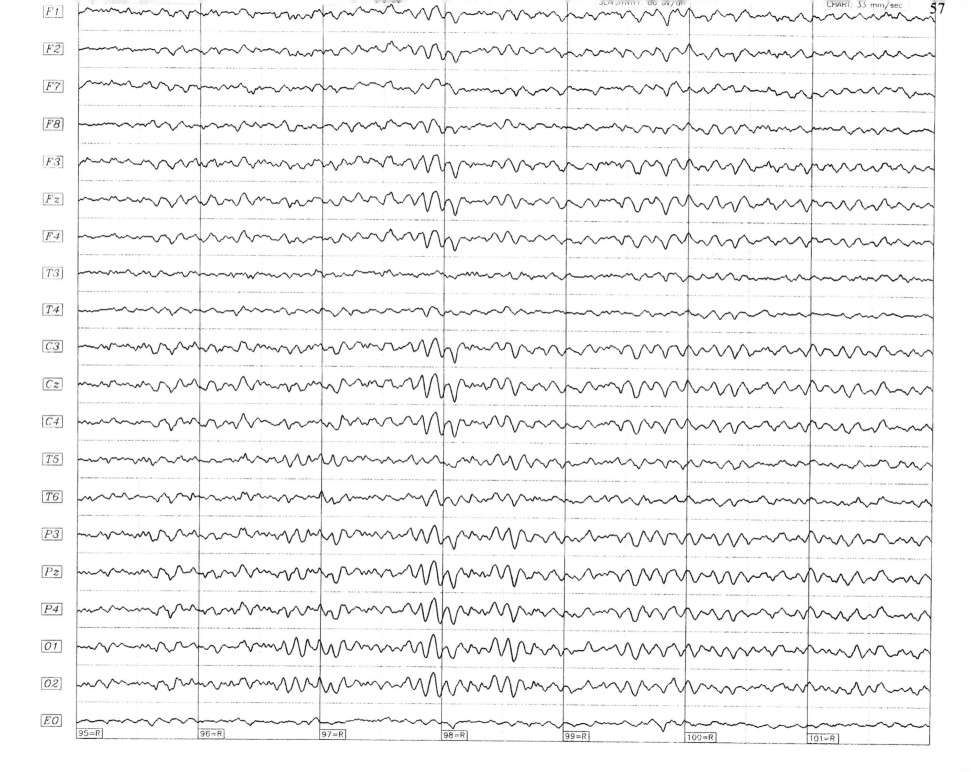

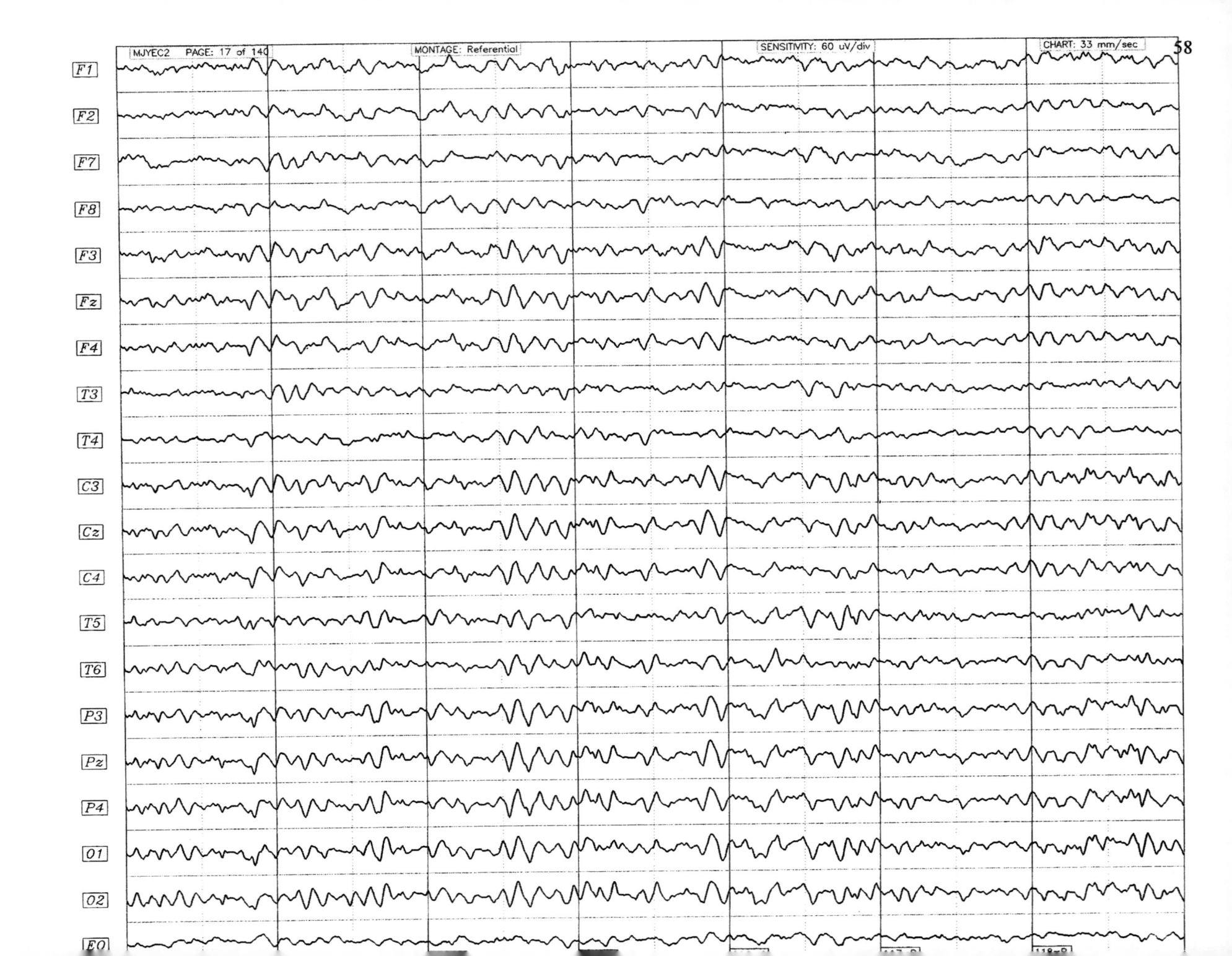

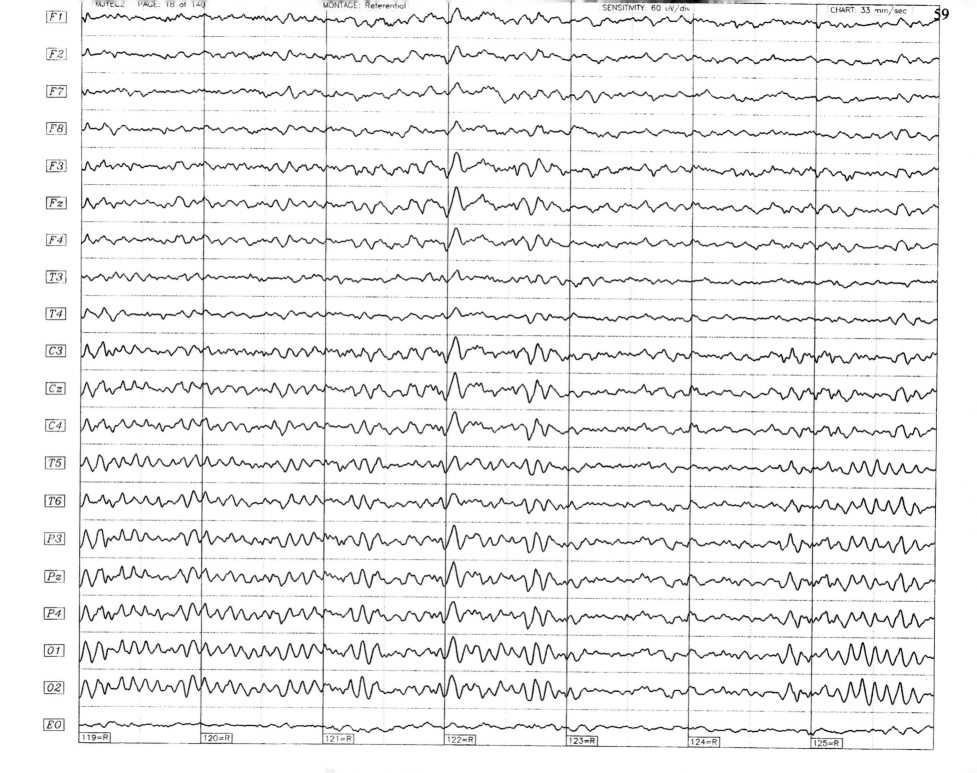

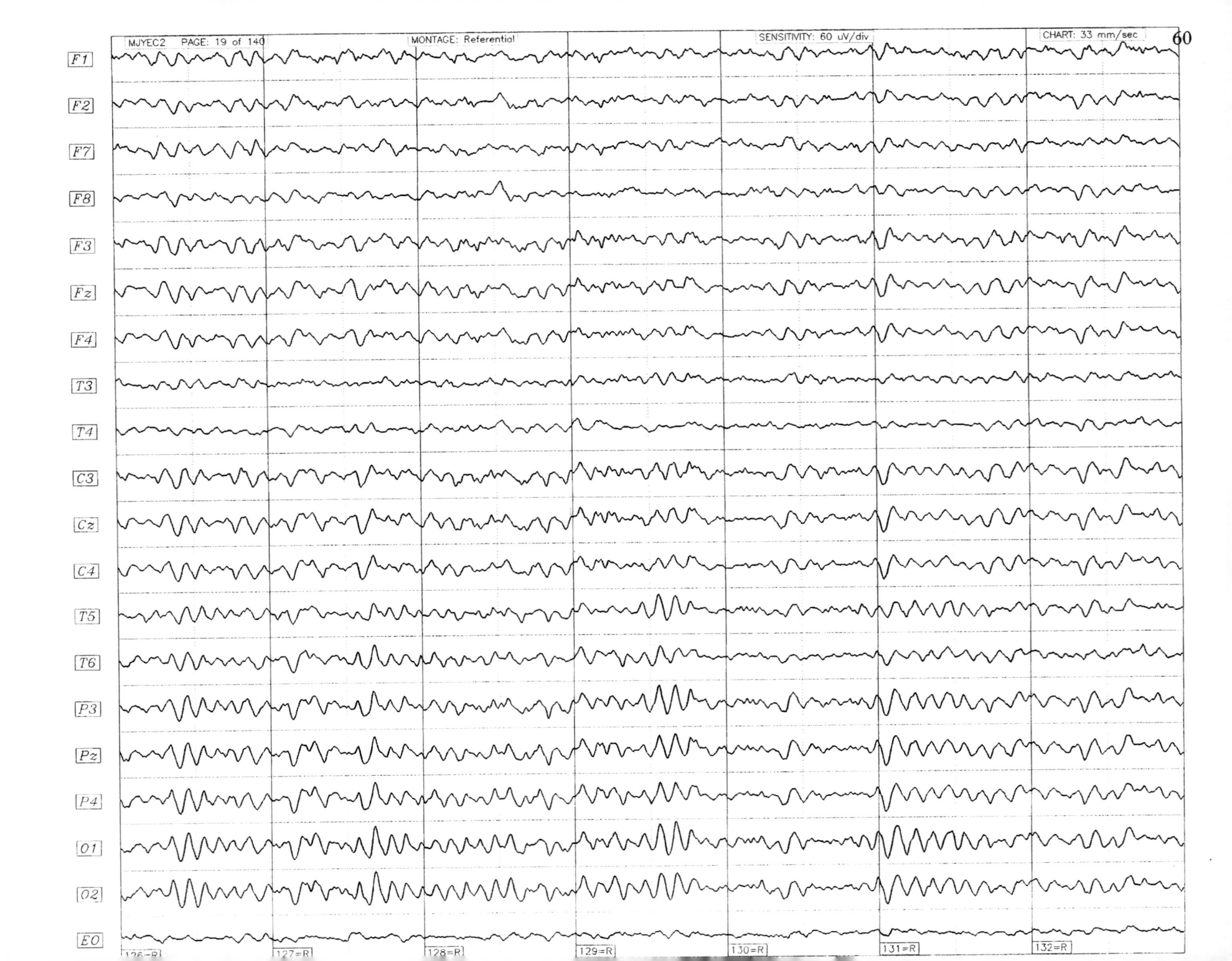

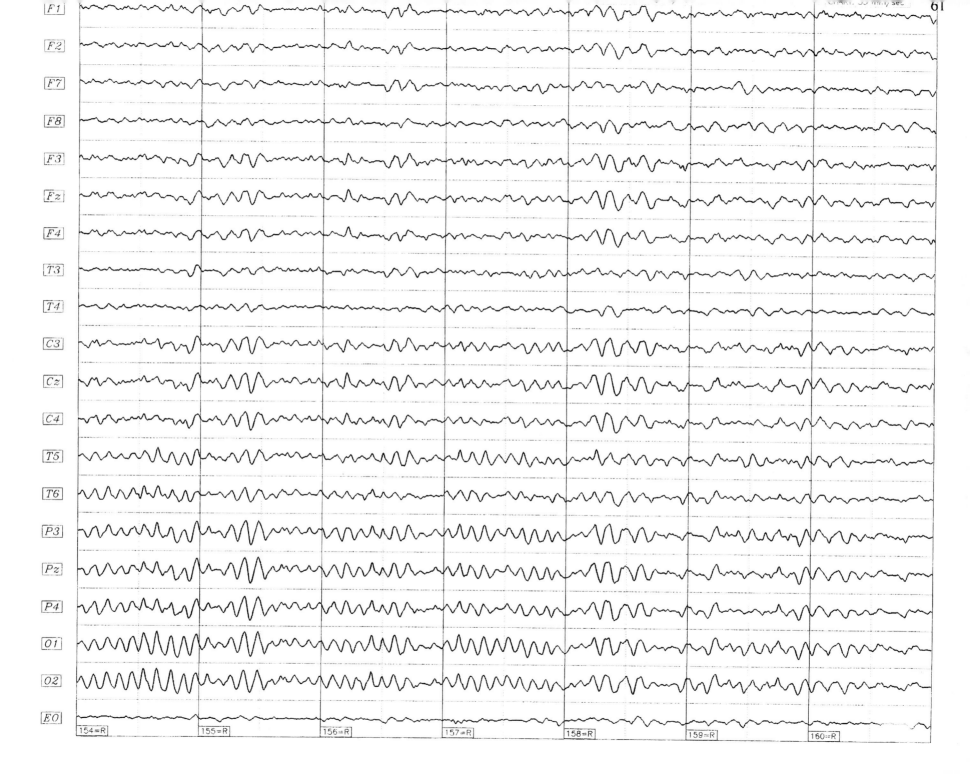

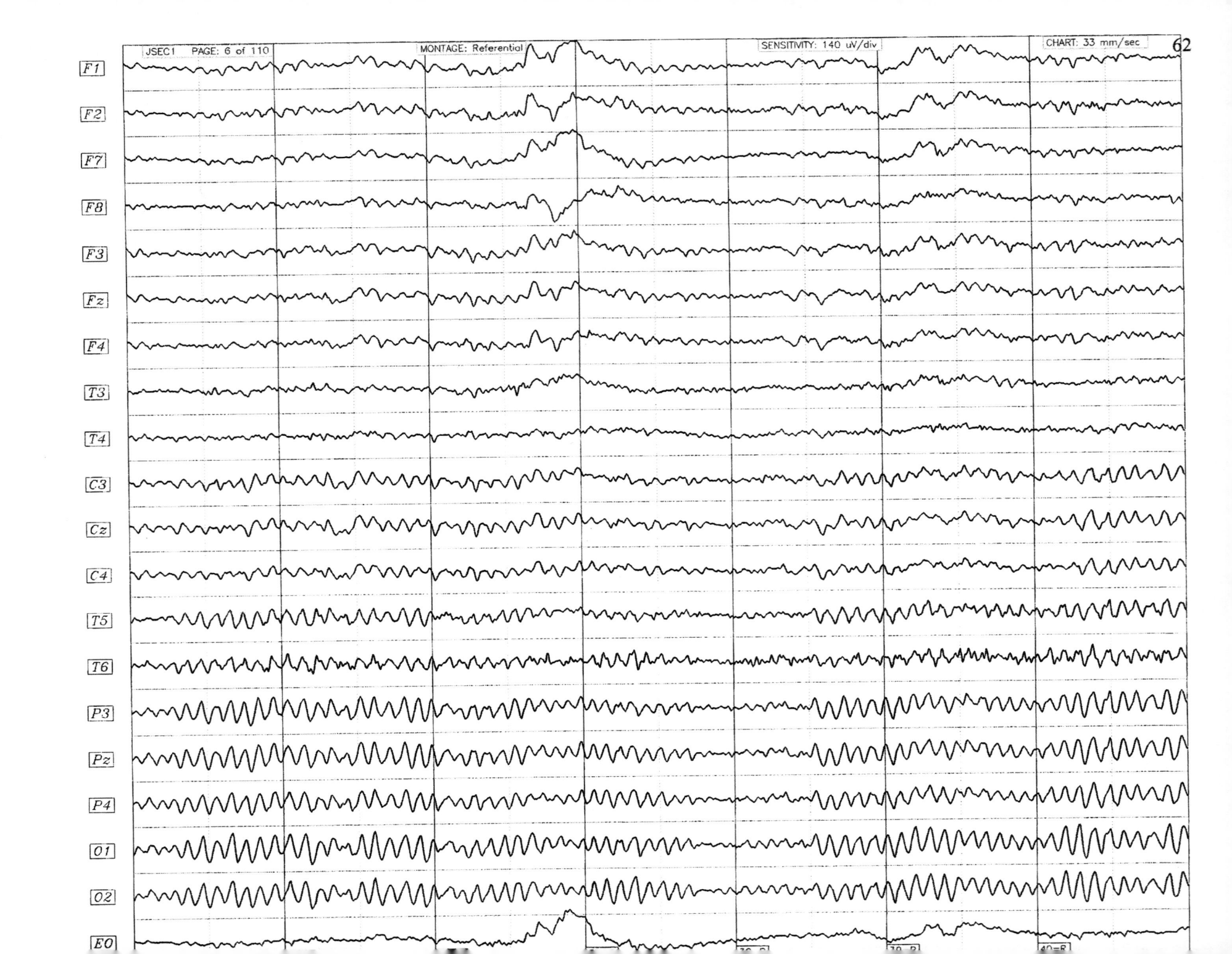

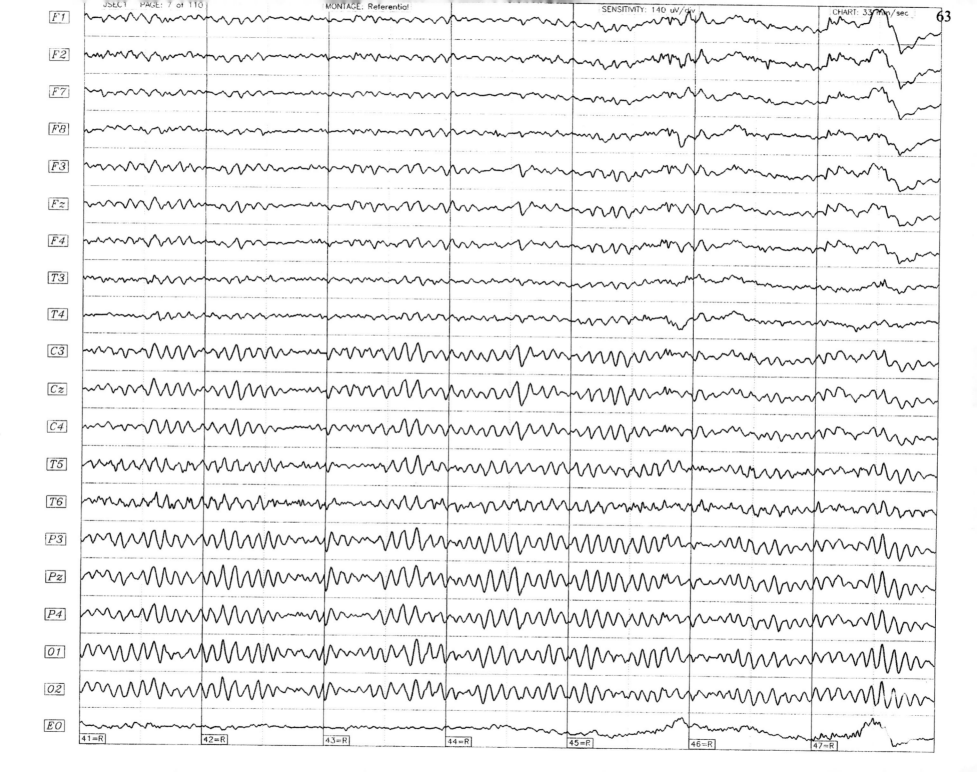

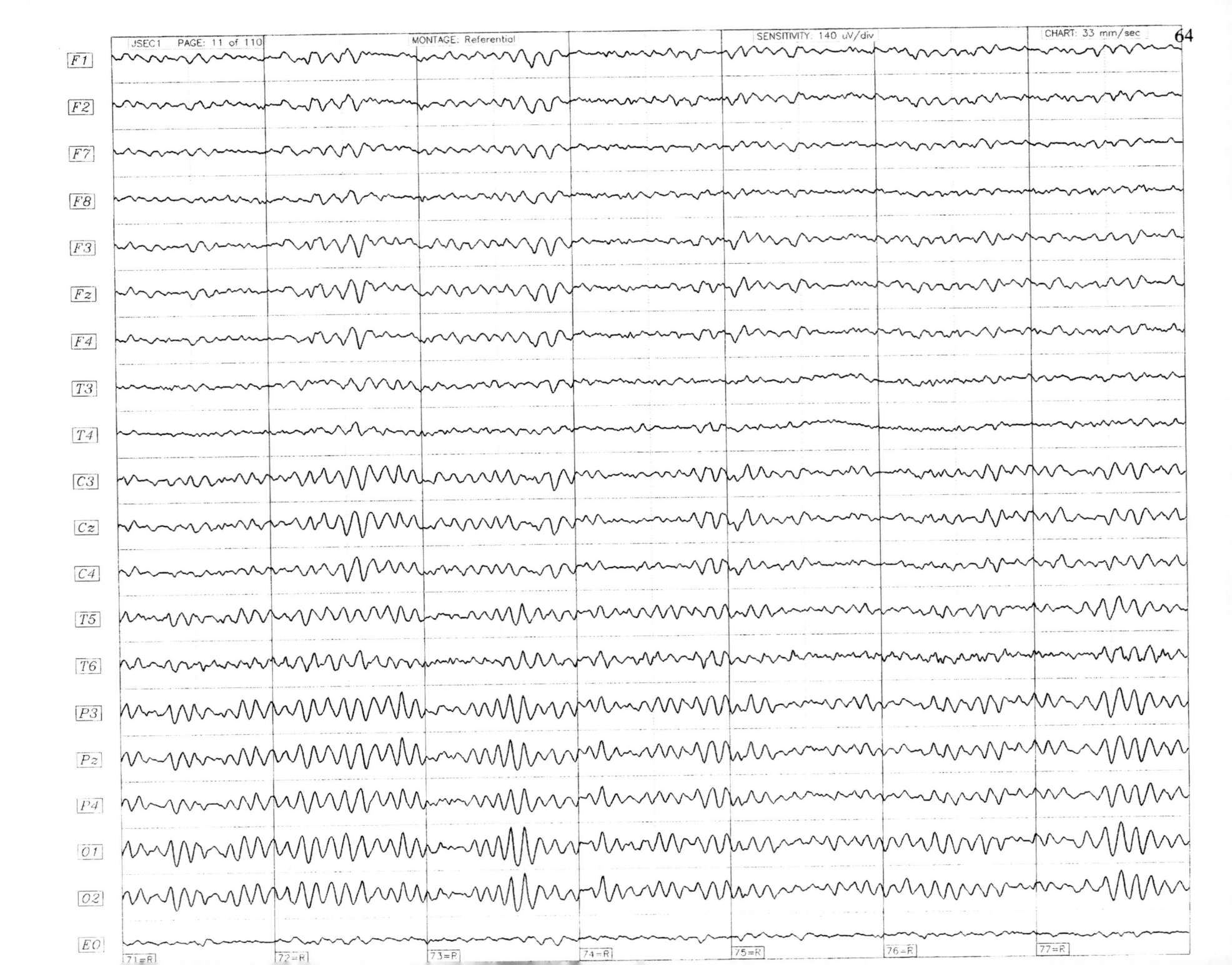

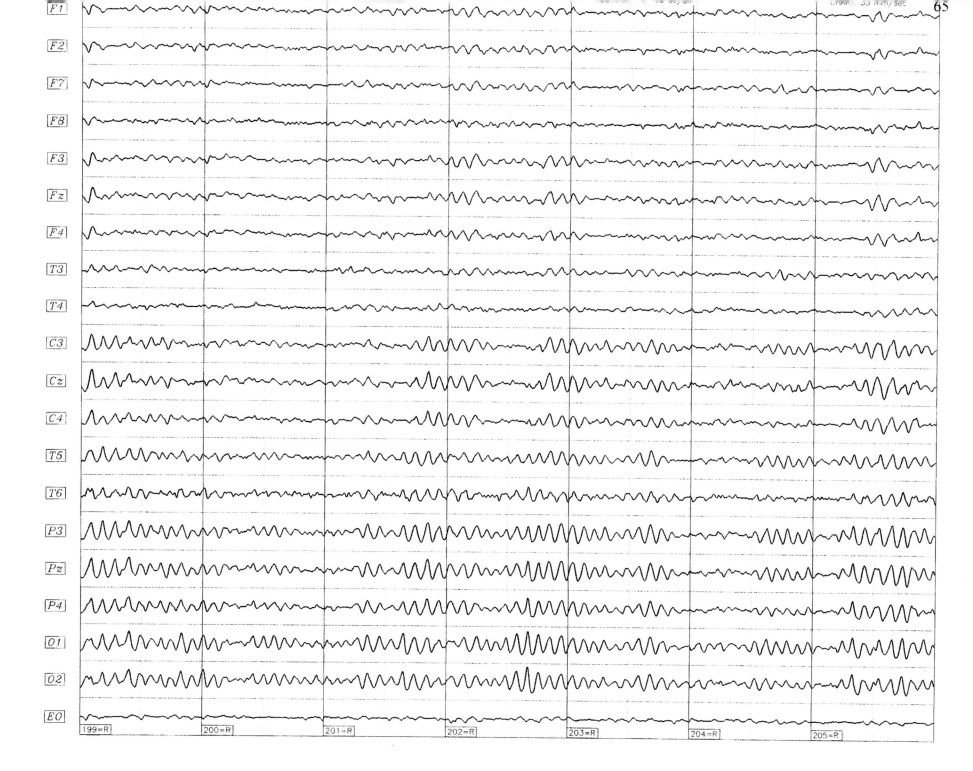

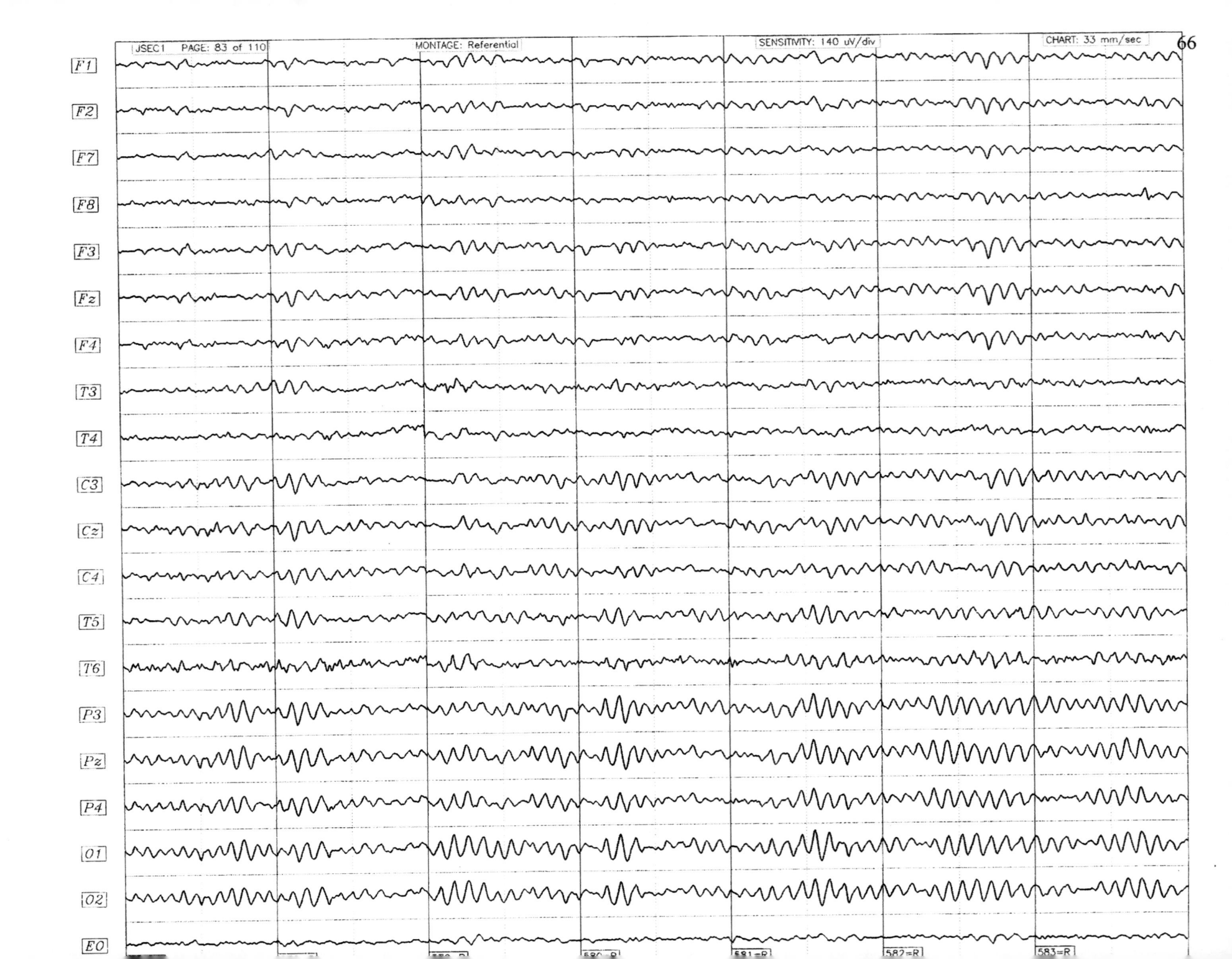

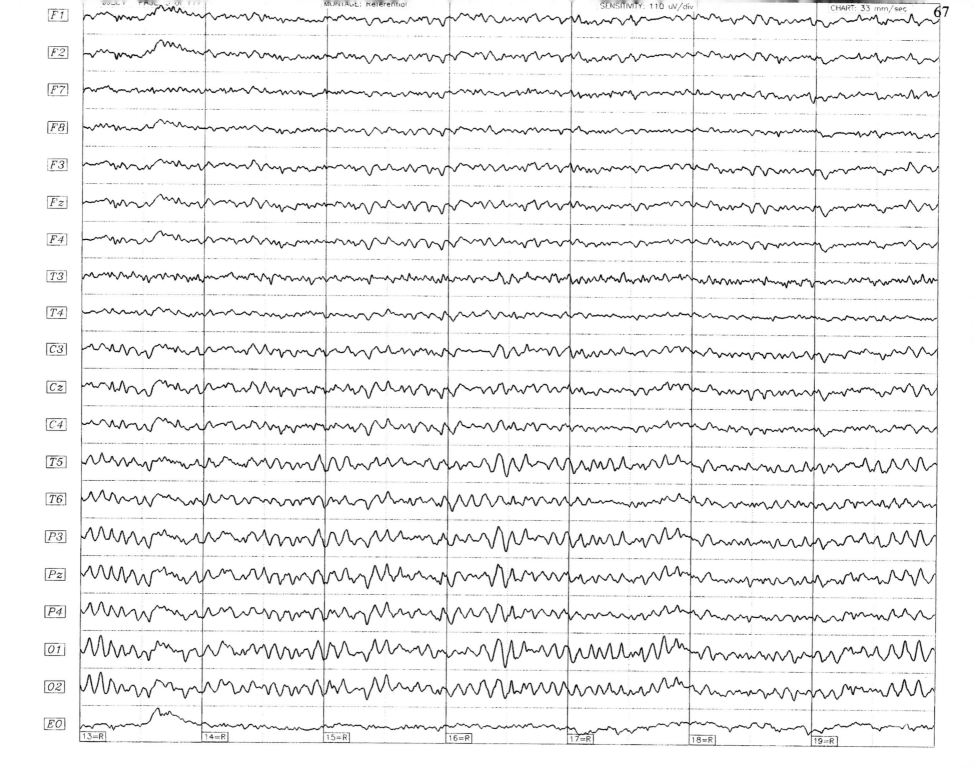

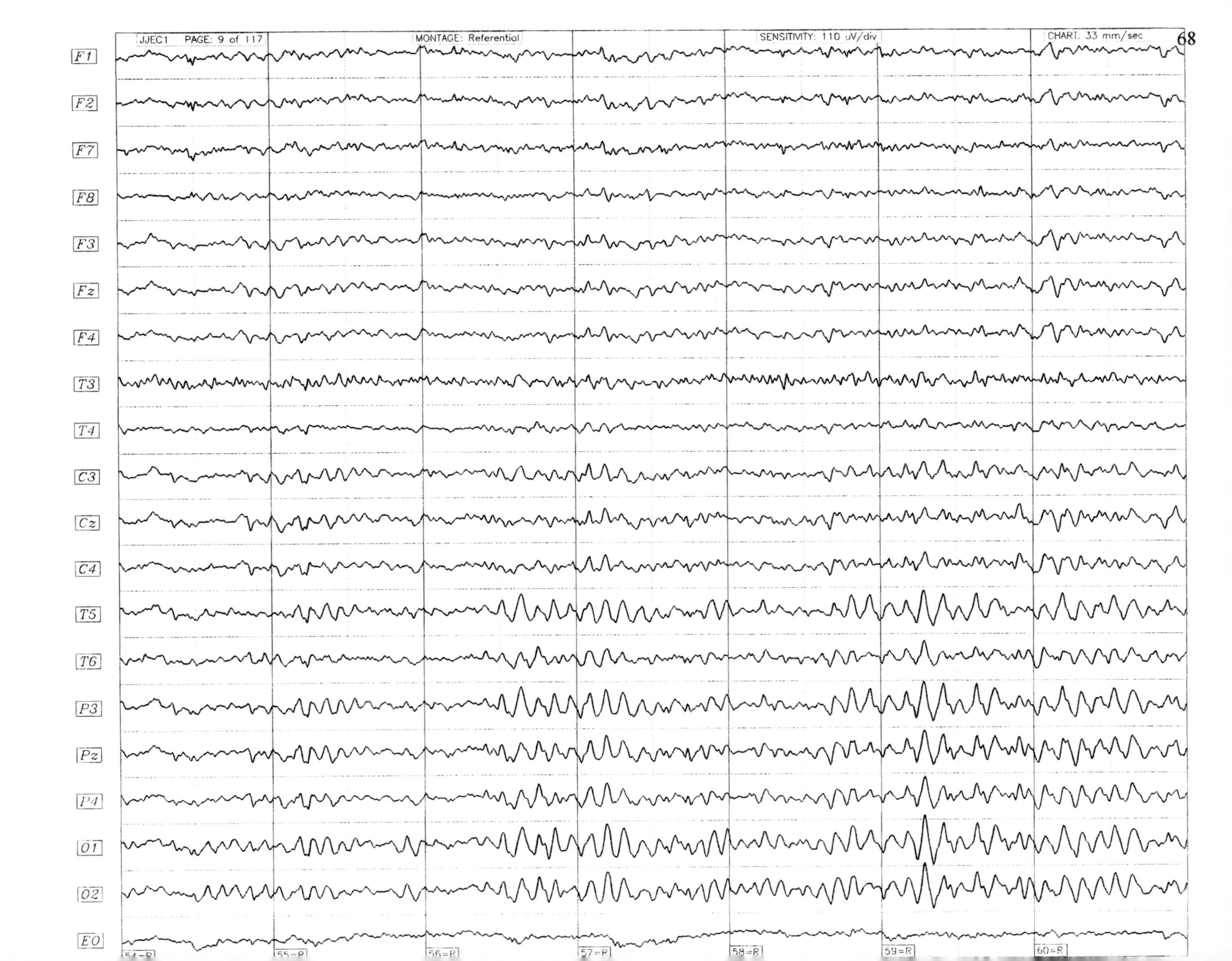

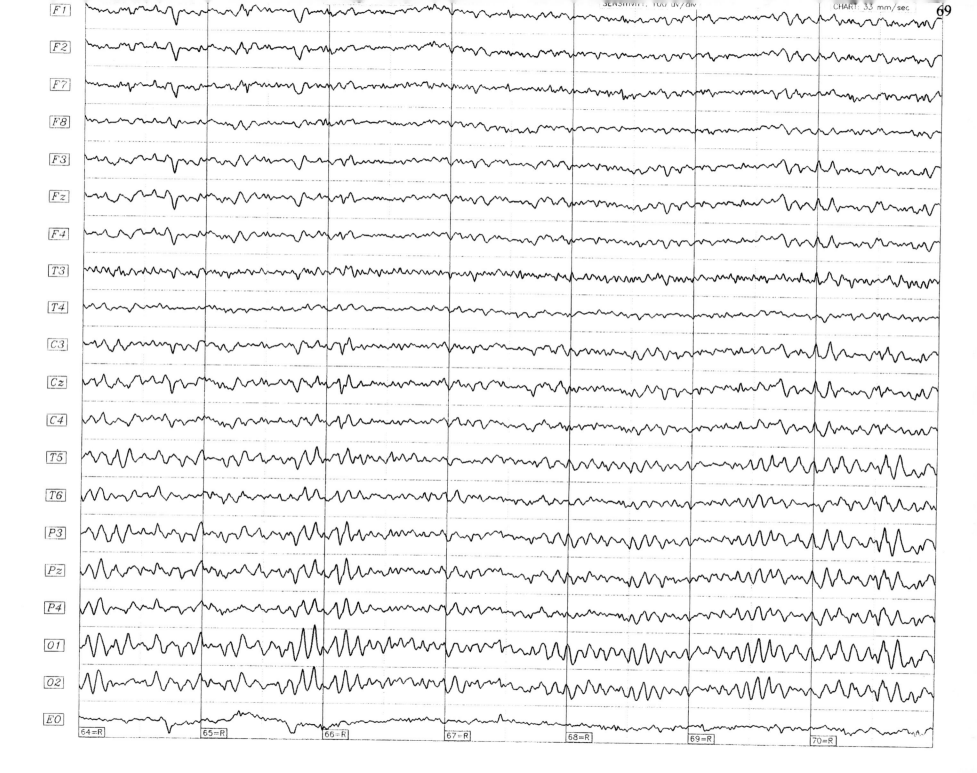

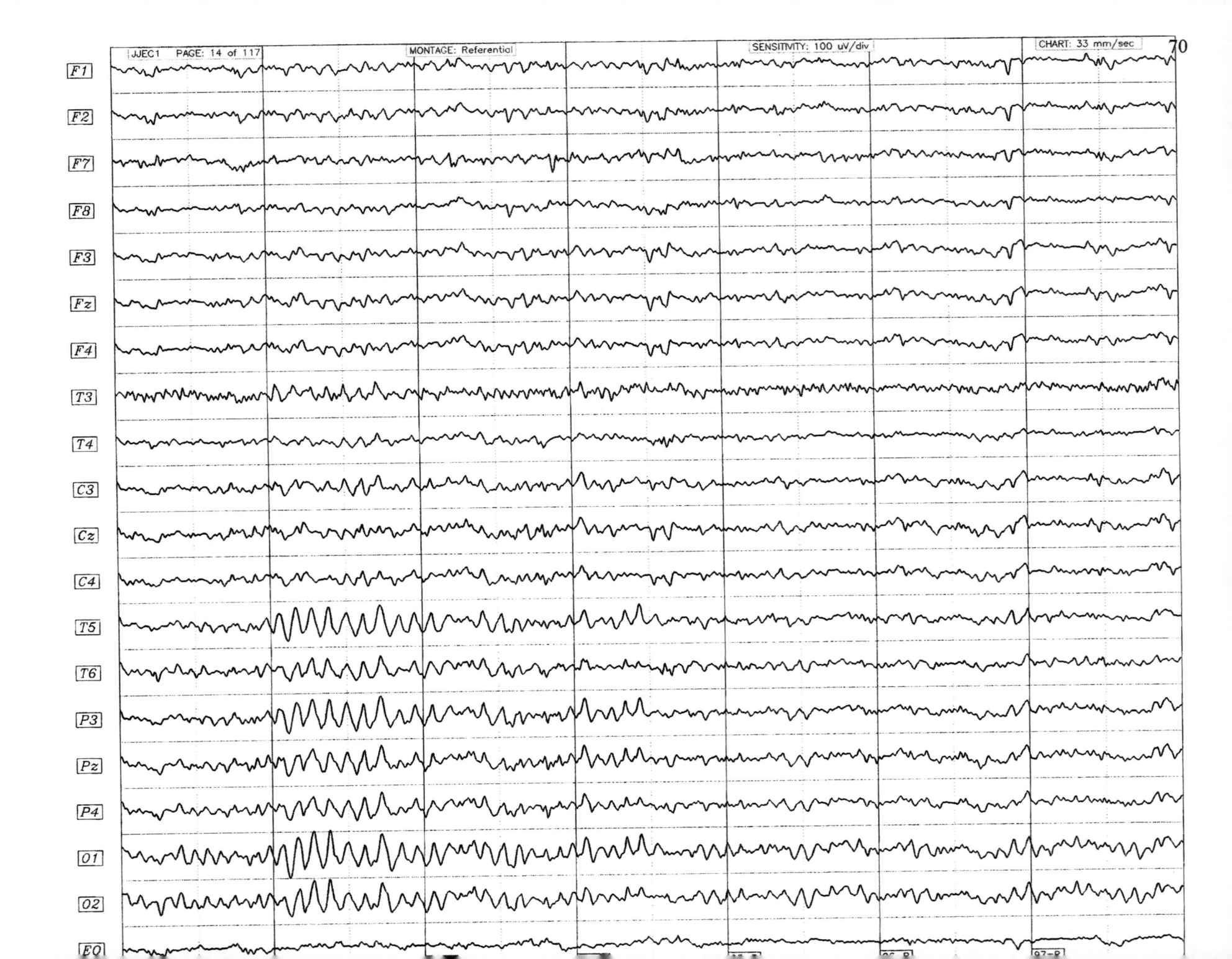

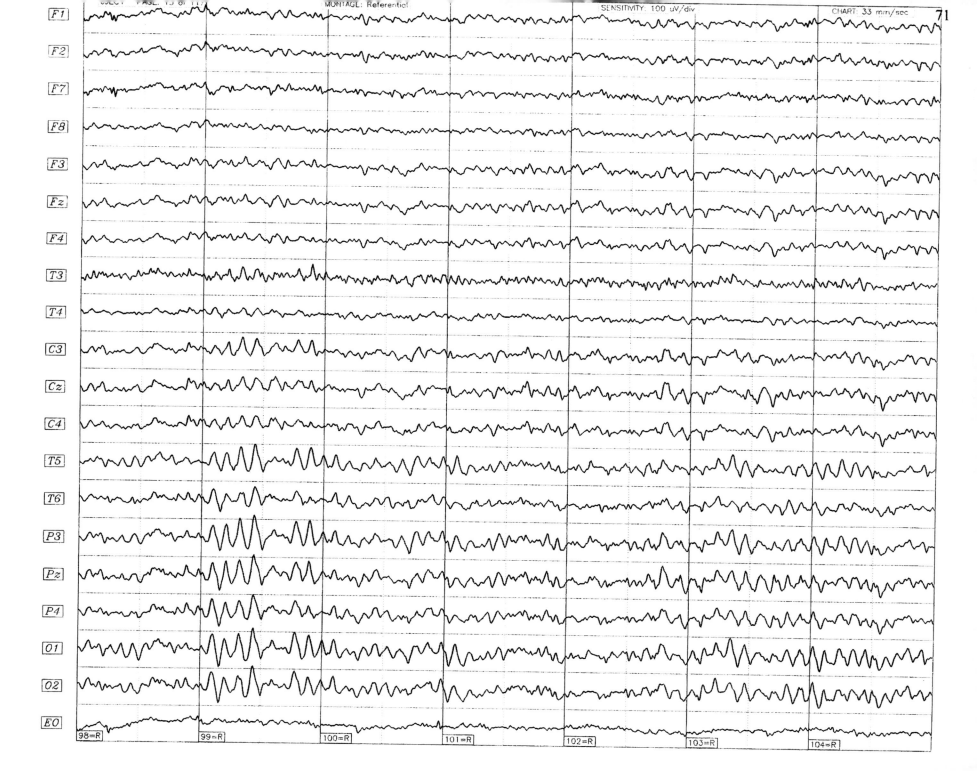

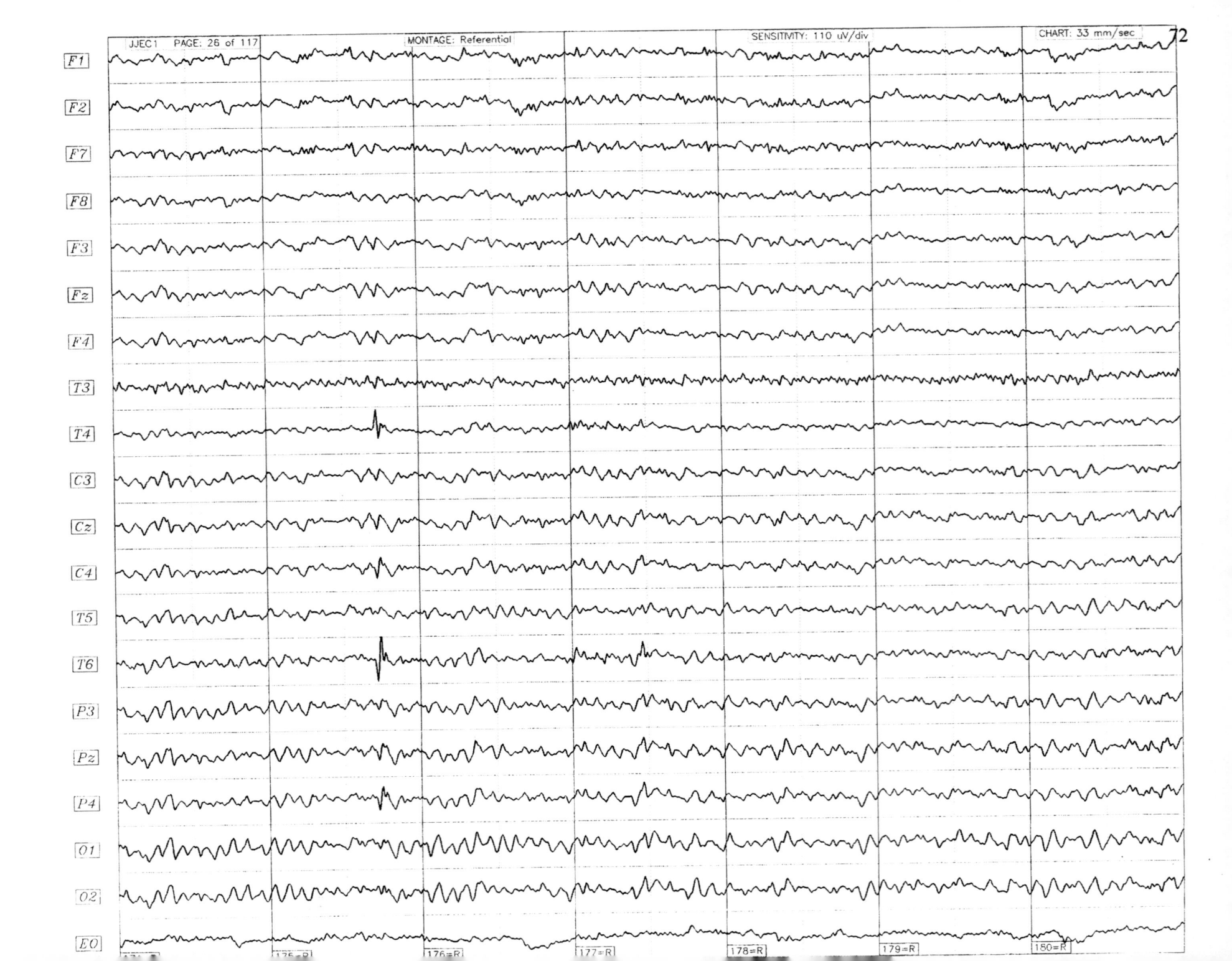

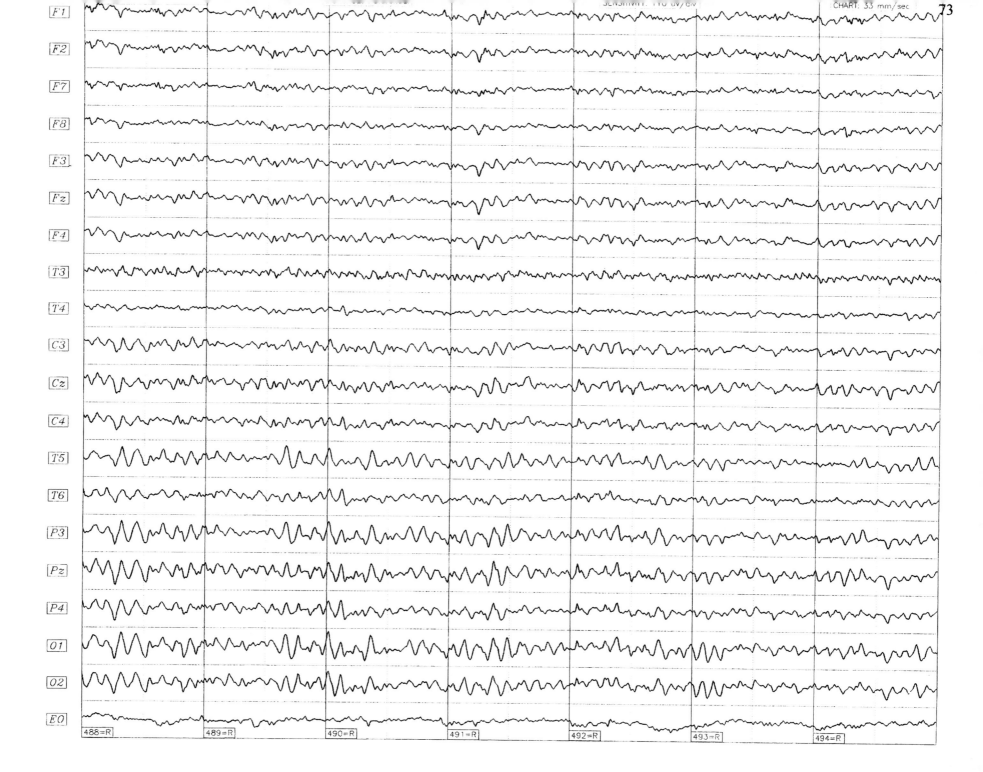

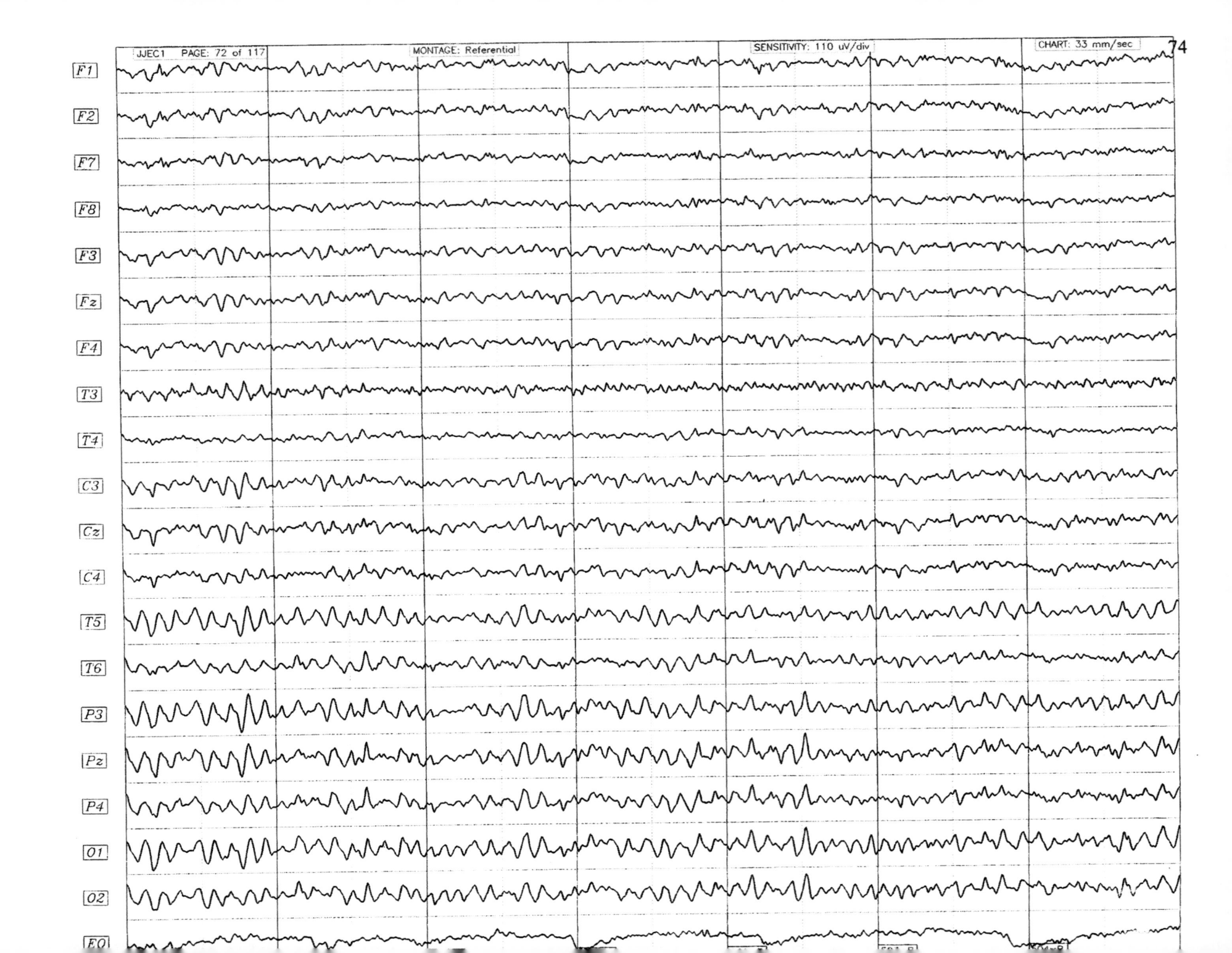

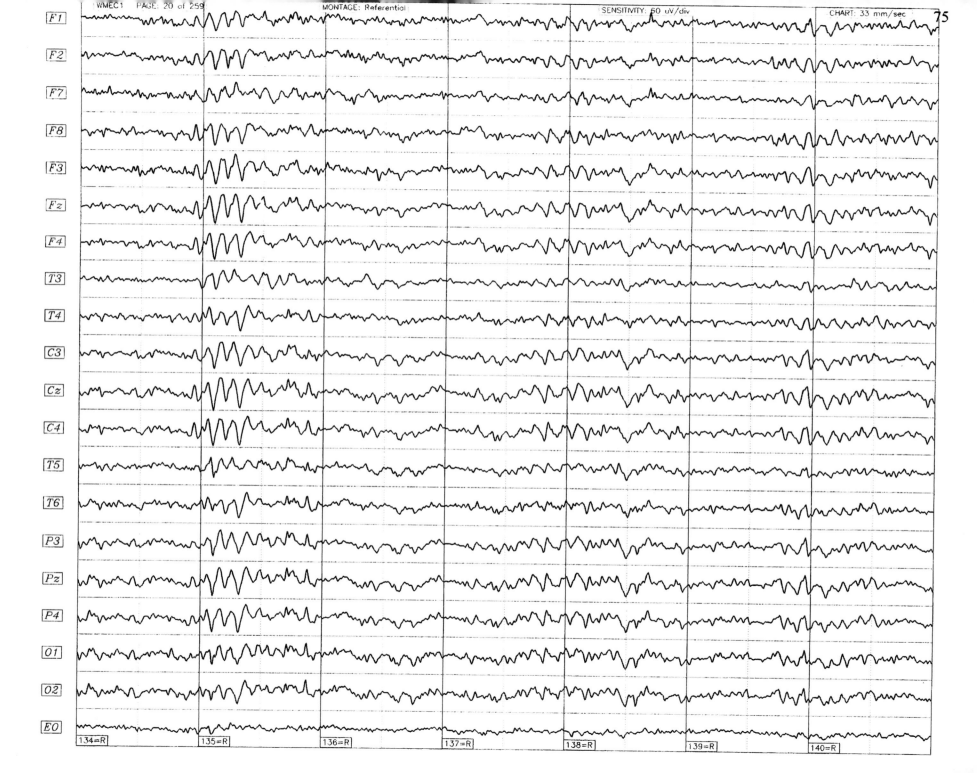

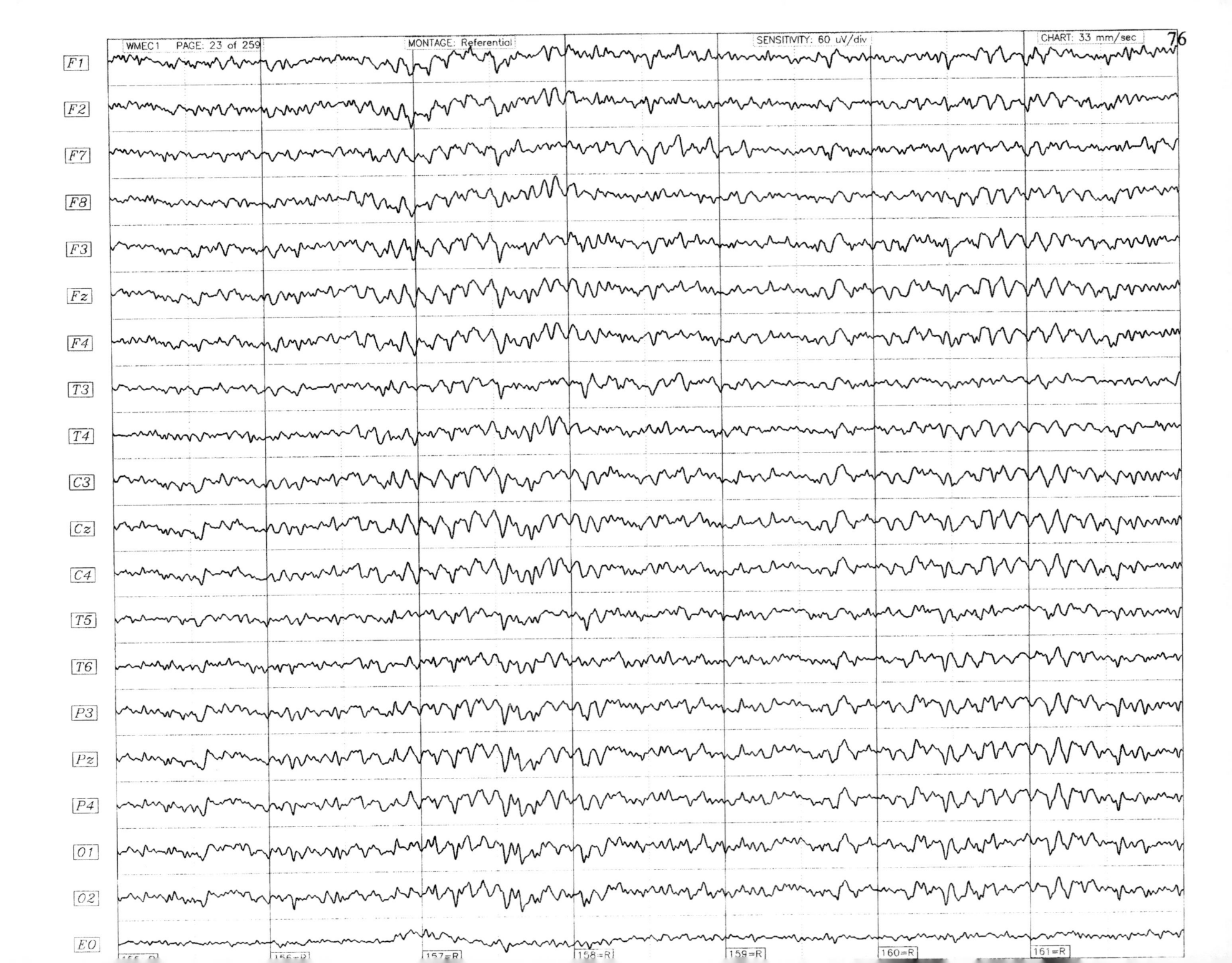

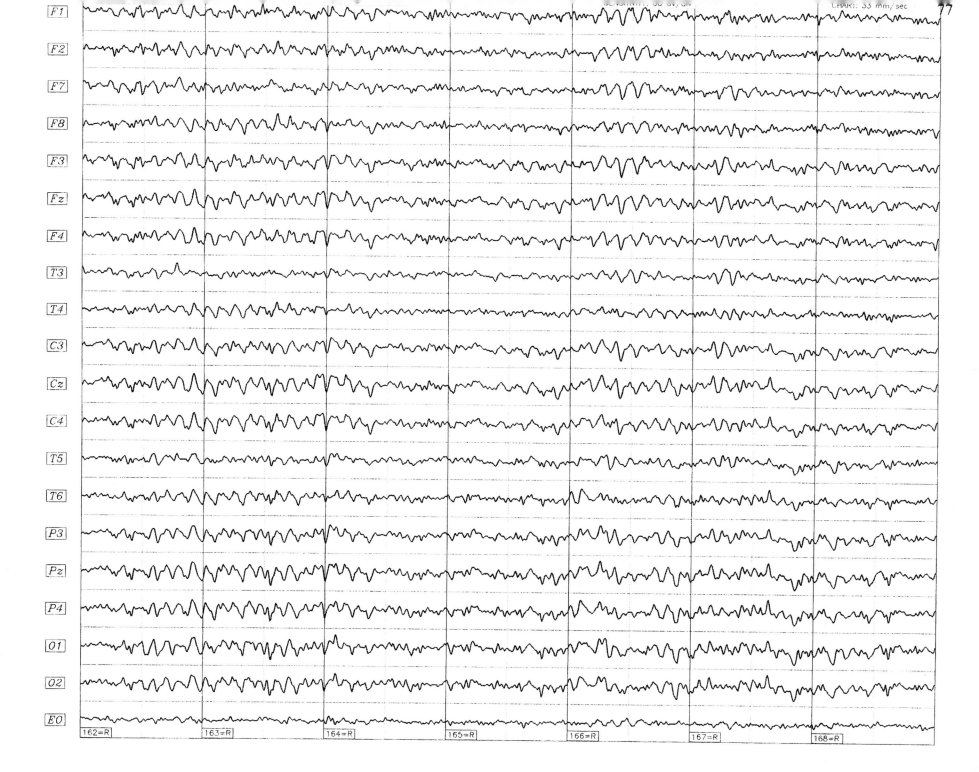

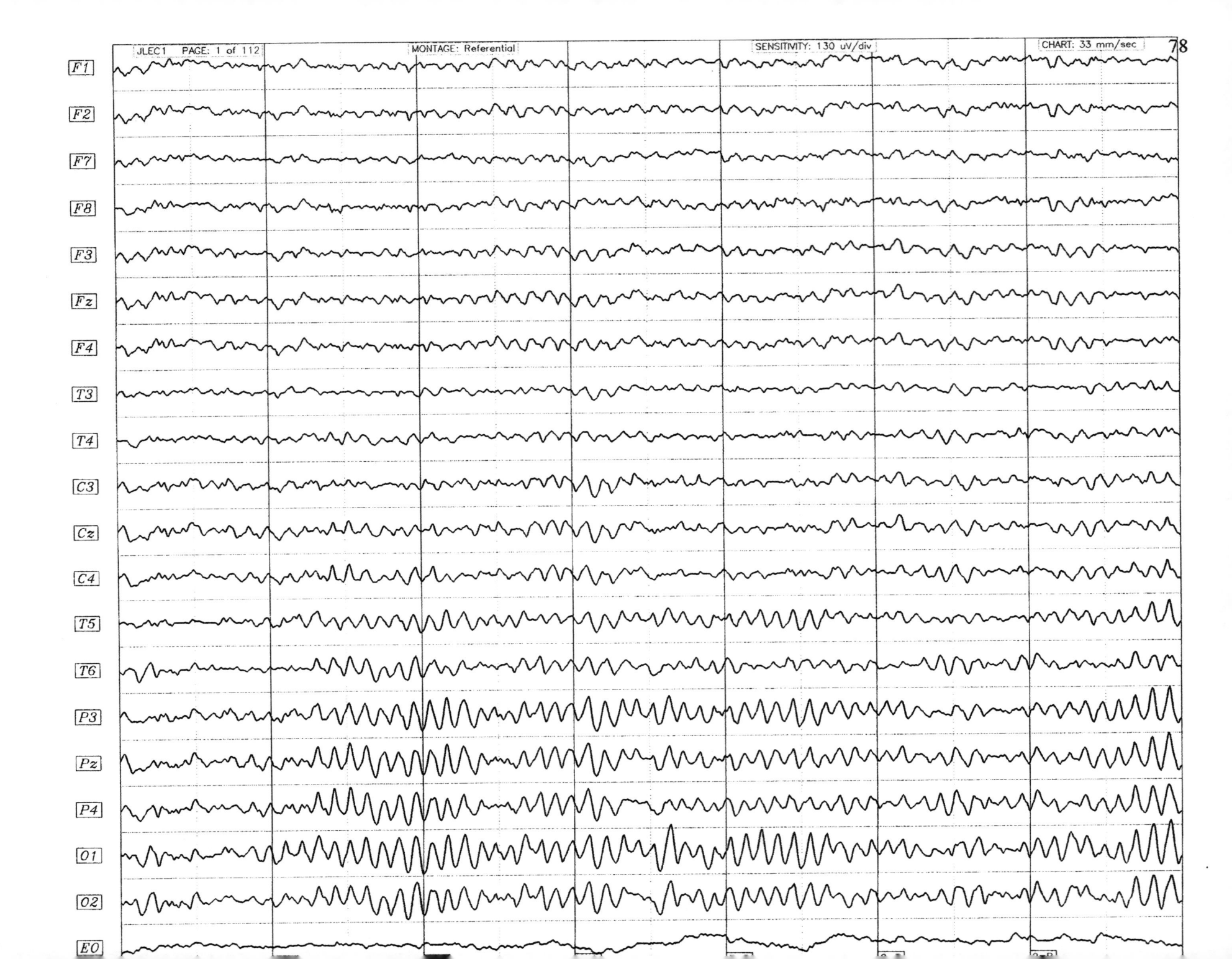

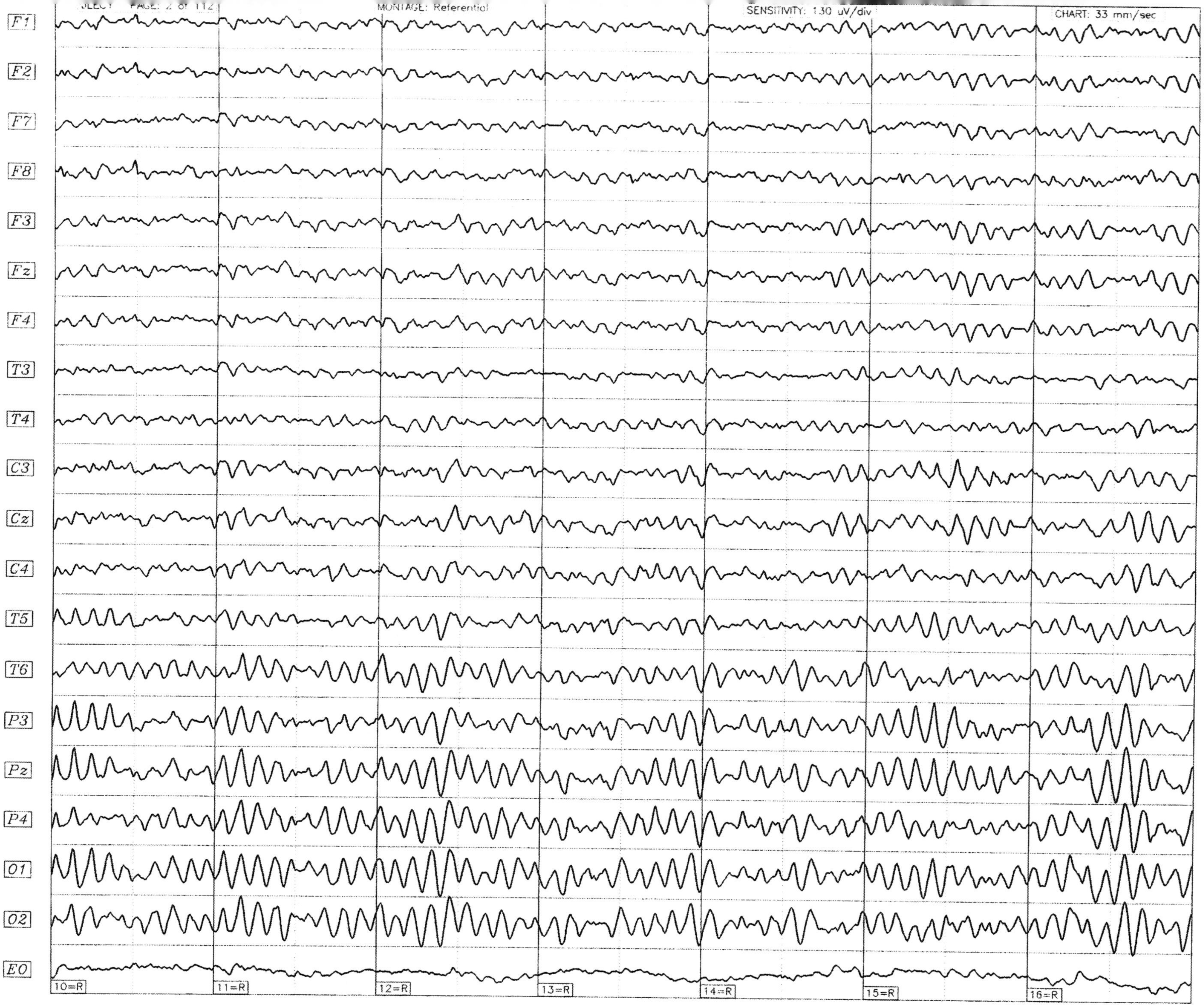
PAGE: 2 of 112
MONTAGE: Referential
SENSITIVITY: 130 uV/div
CHART: 33 mm/sec
F1
F2
F7
F8
F3
Fz
F4
T3
T4
C3
Cz
C4
T5
T6
P3
Pz
P4
O1
O2
EO
10=R
11=R
12=R
13=R
14=R
15=R
16=R

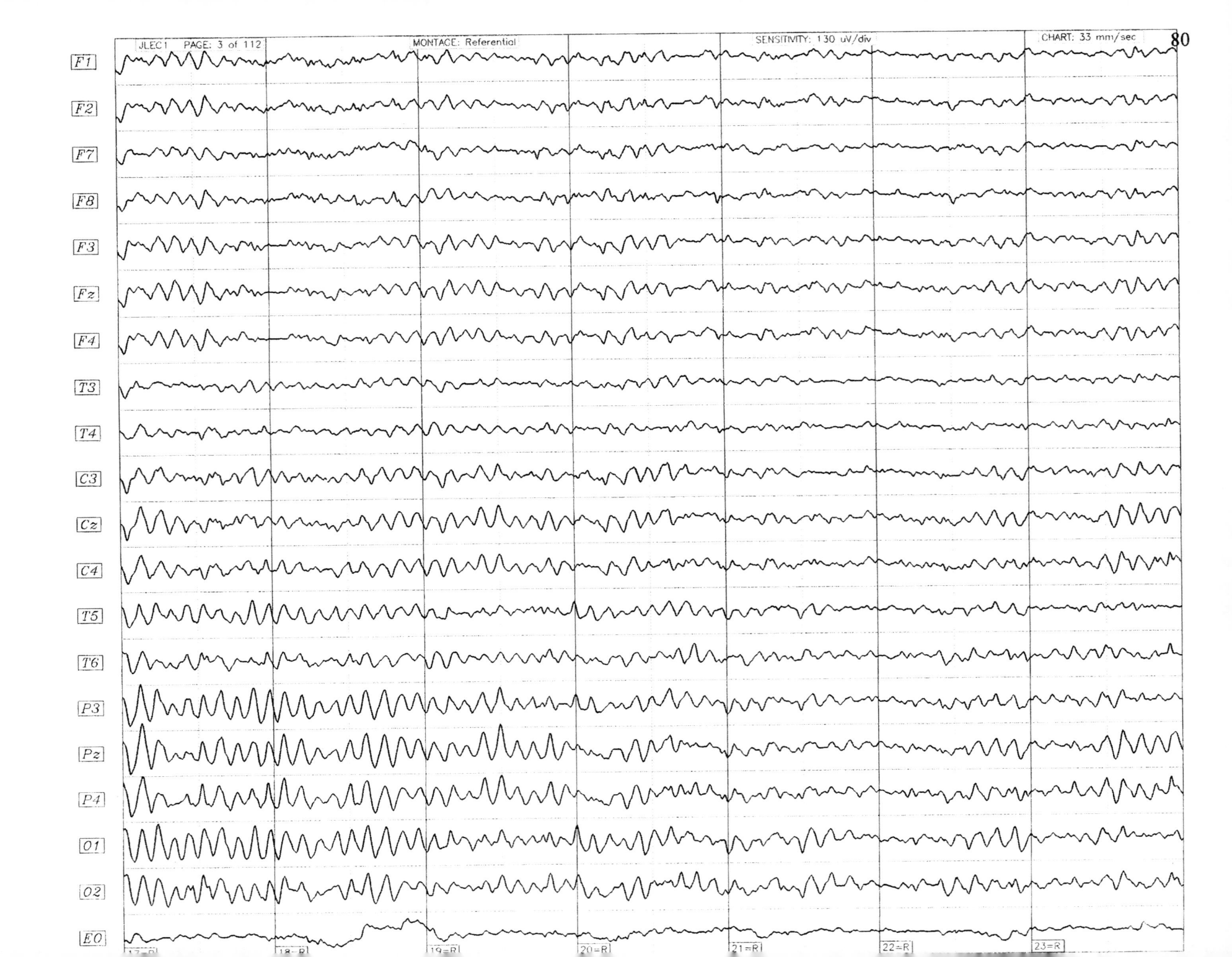

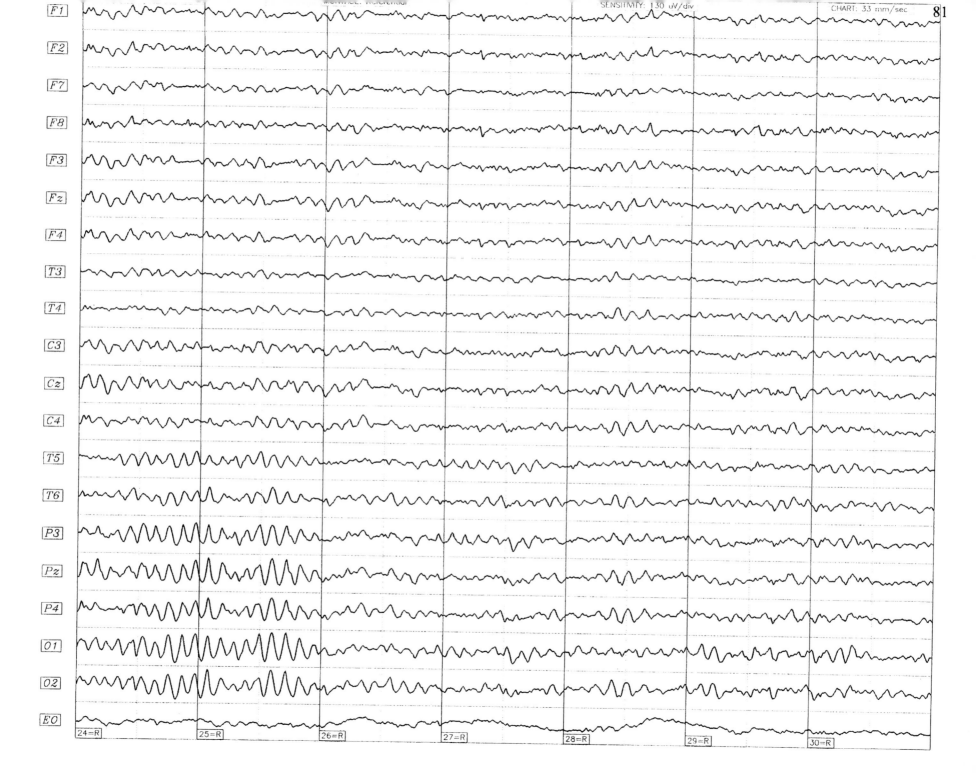

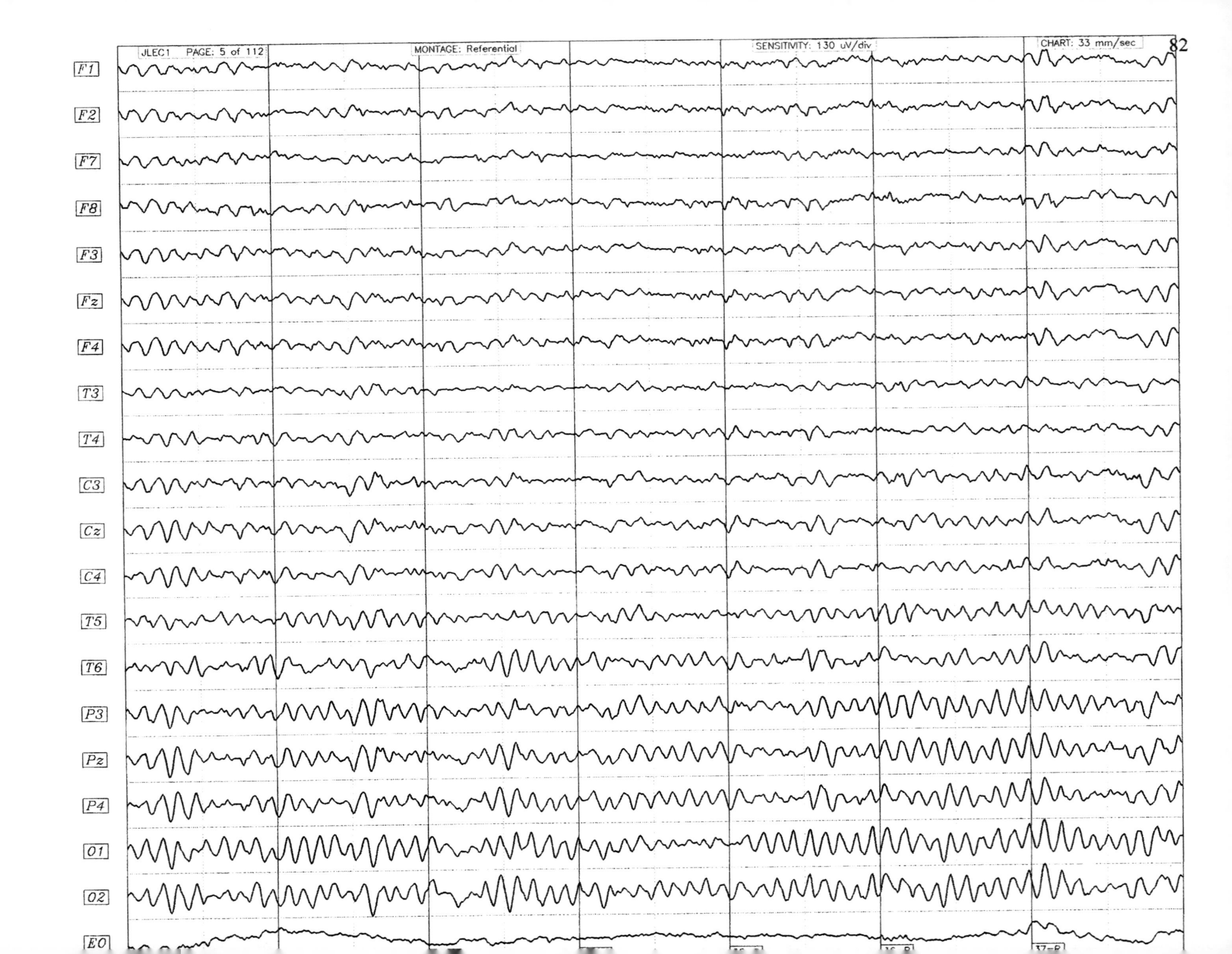

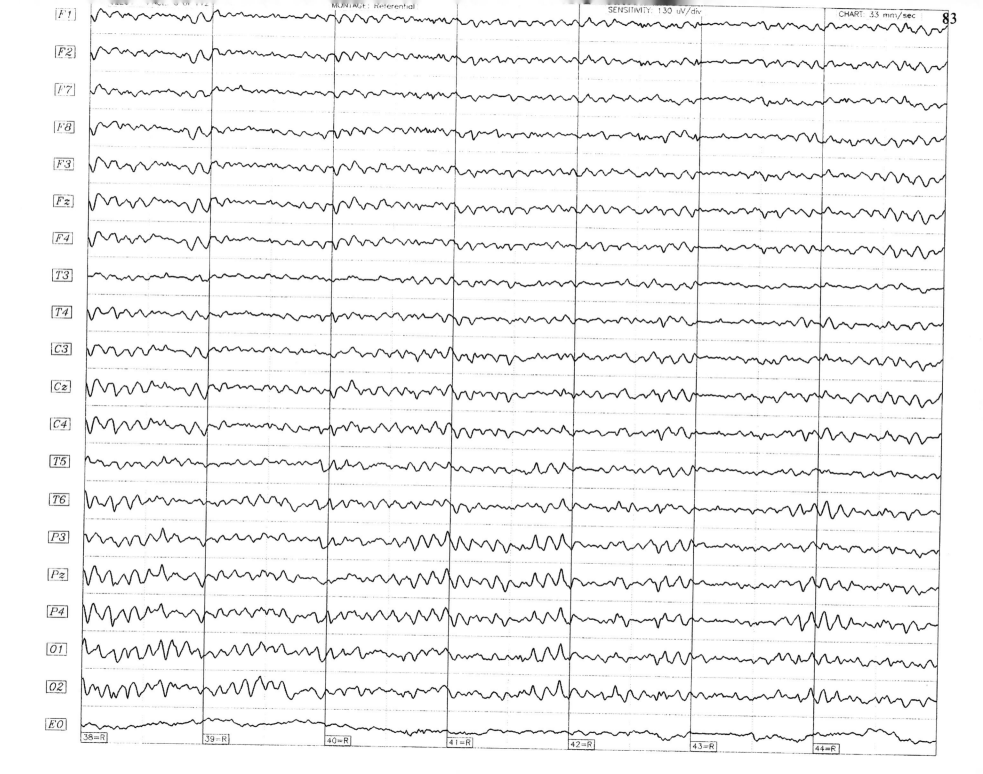

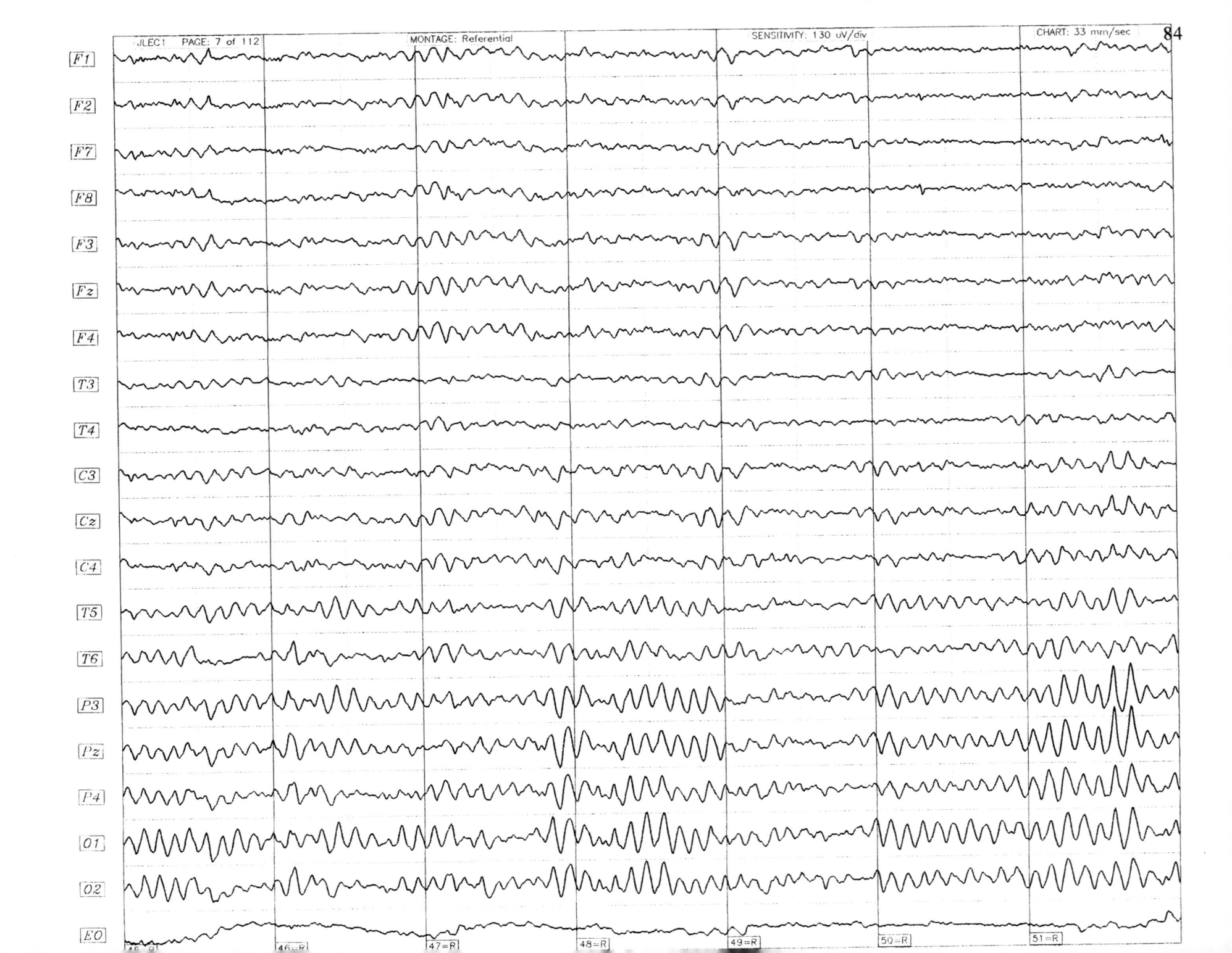

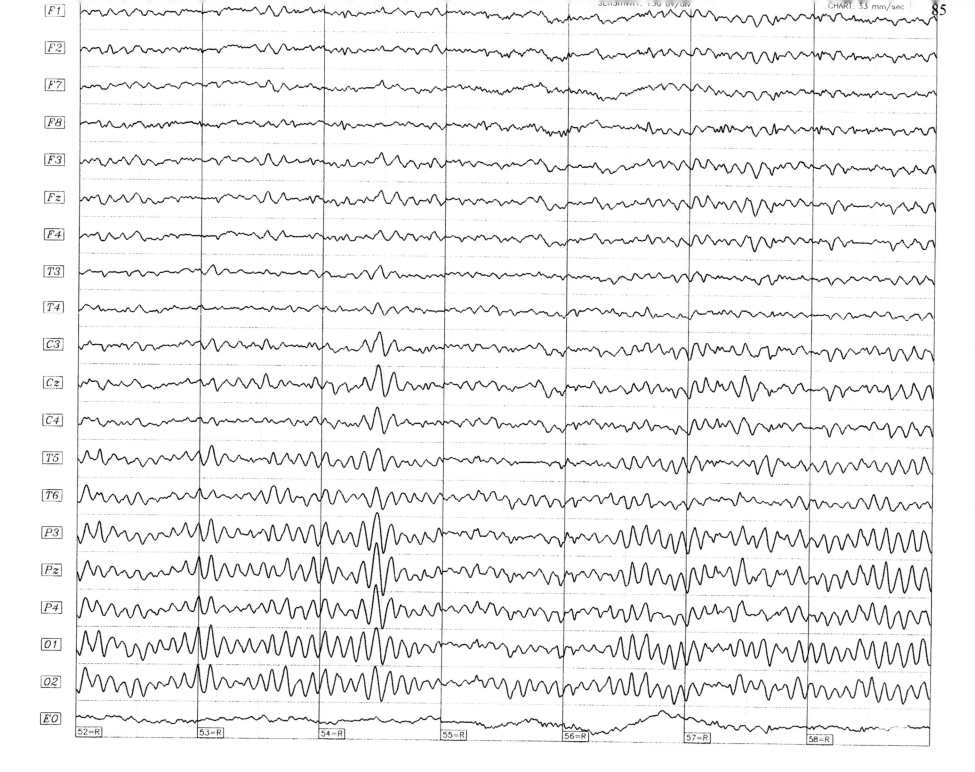

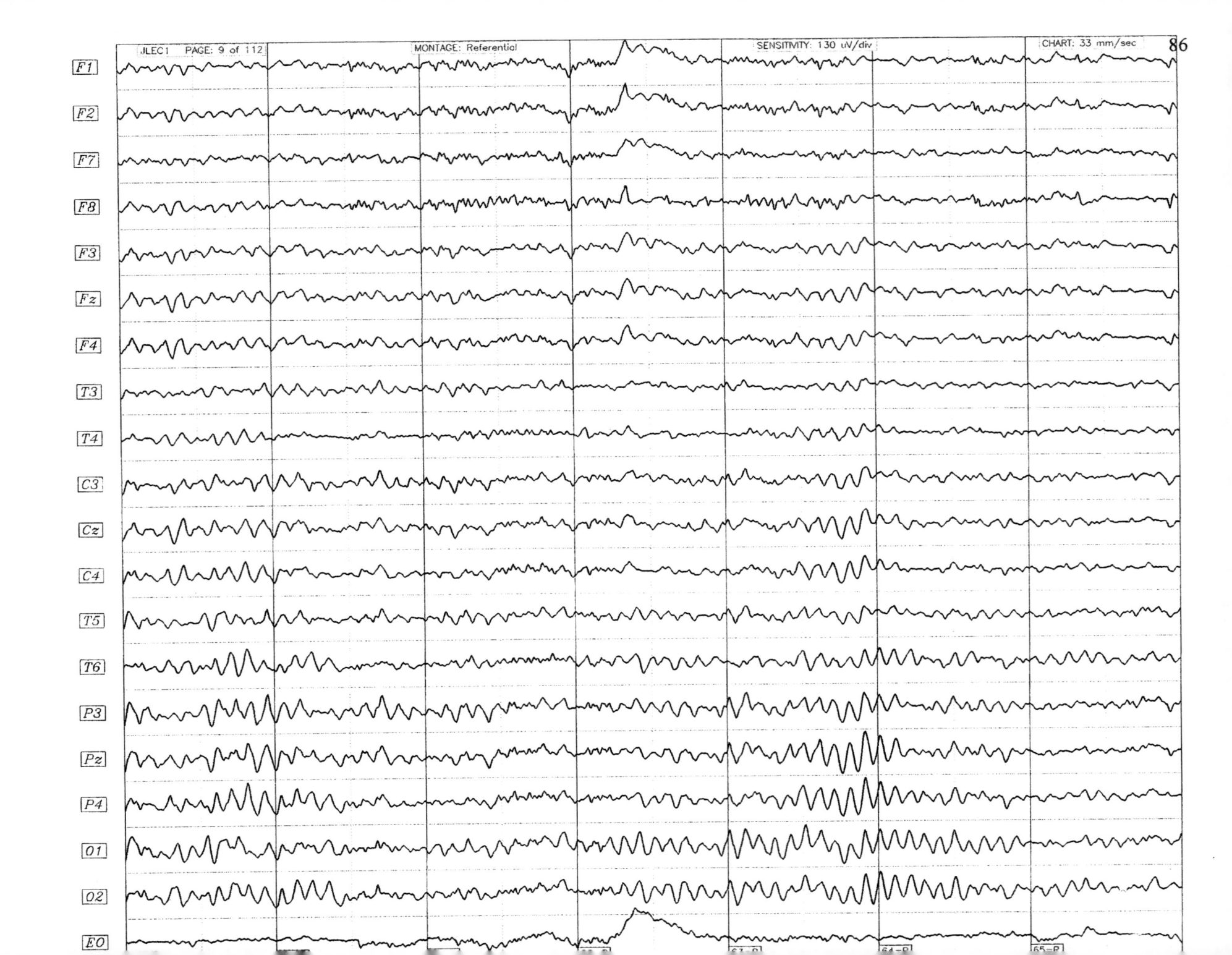

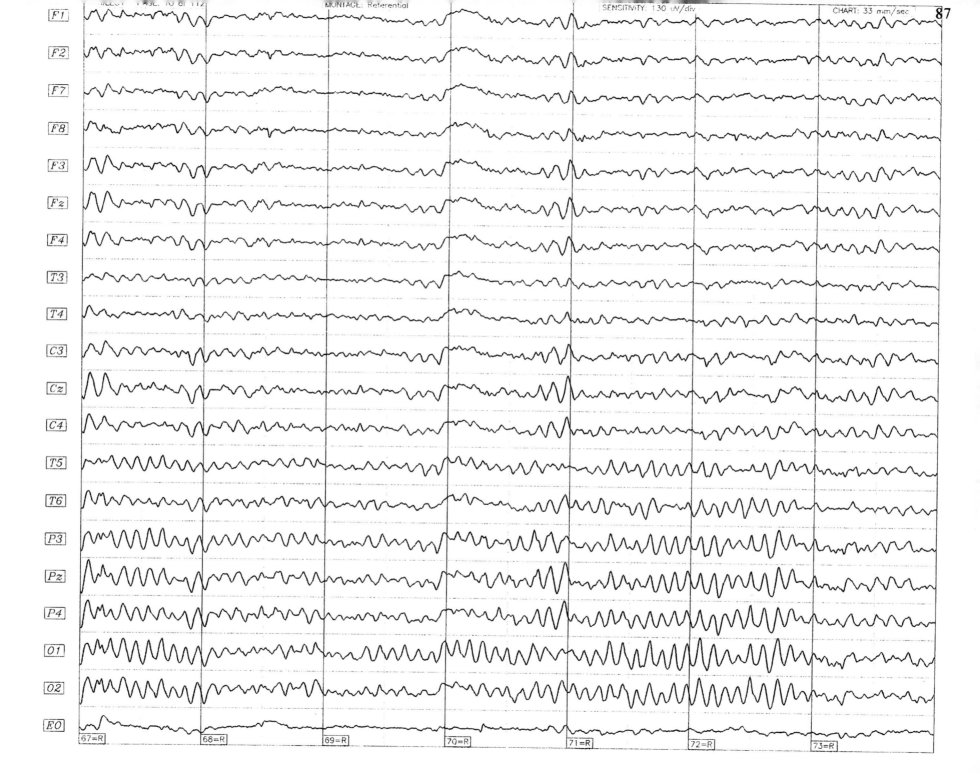

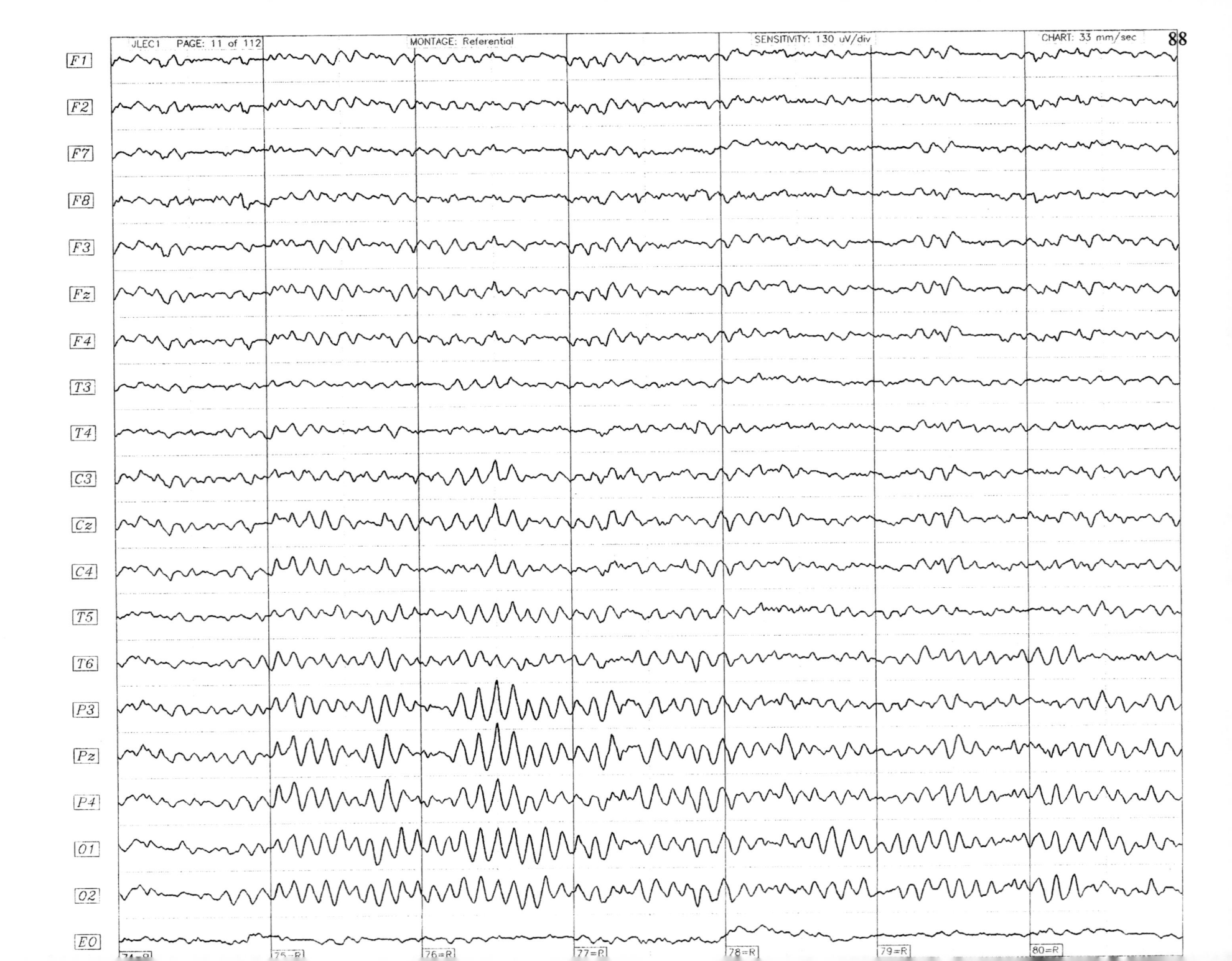

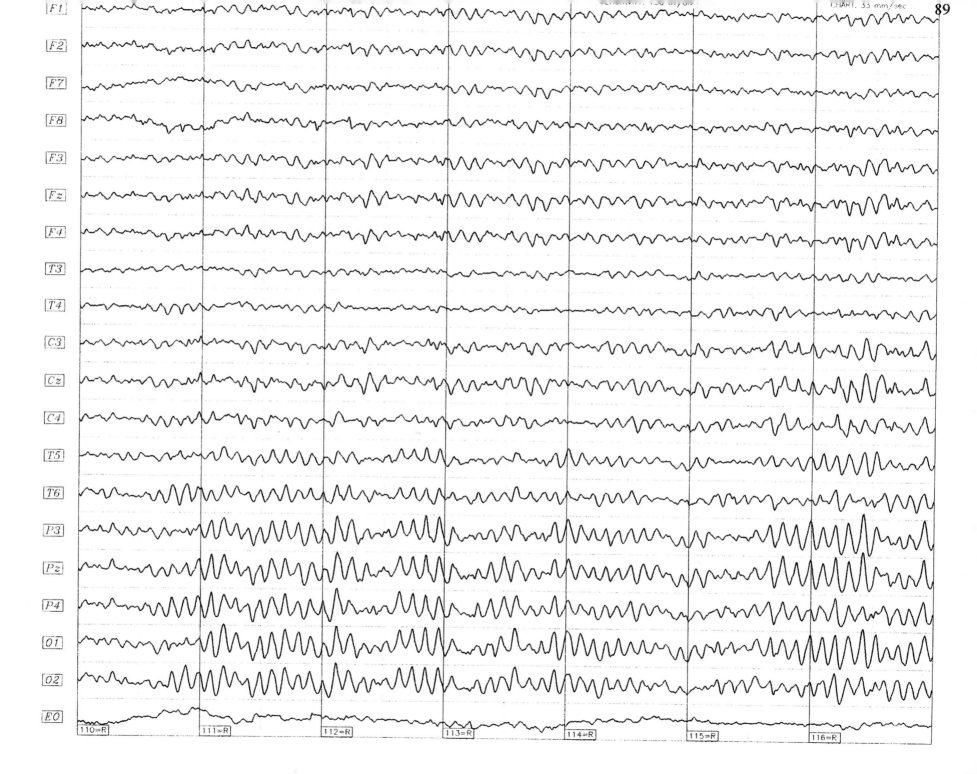

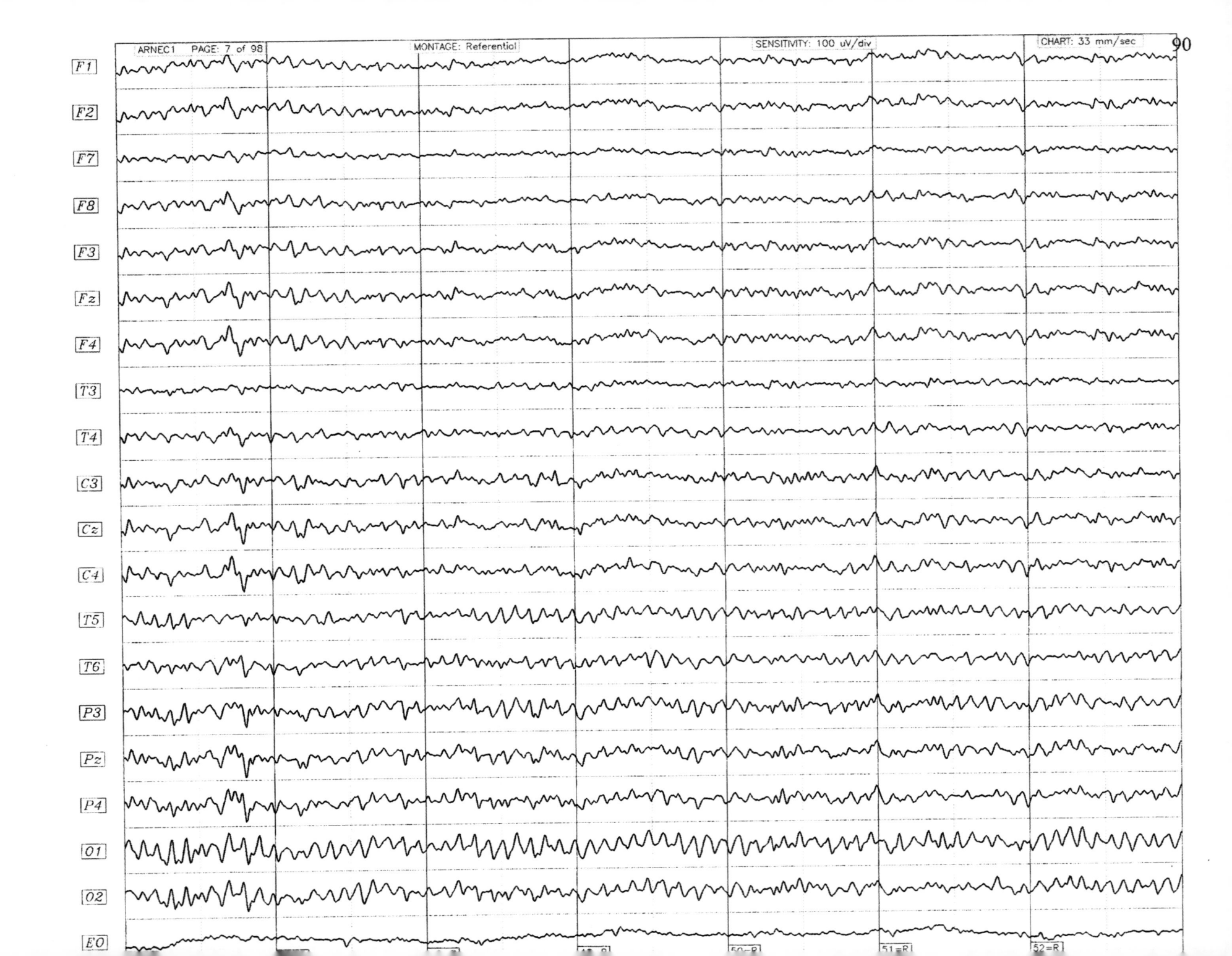

MONTAGE: Referential

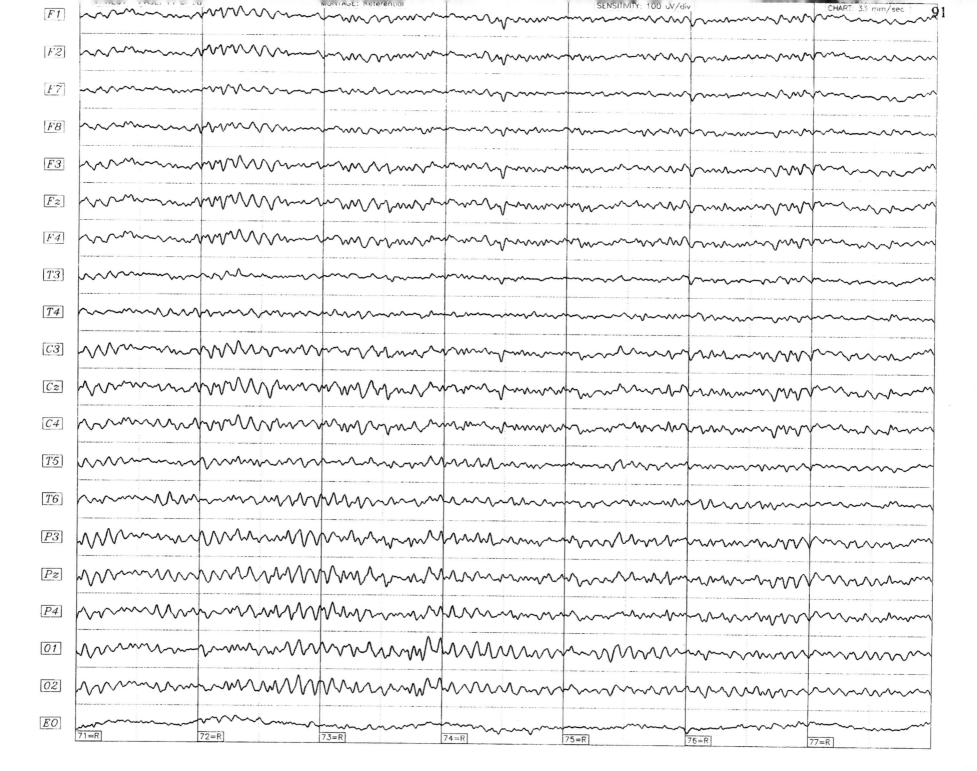

| F1 |
| F2 |
| F7 |
| F8 |
| F3 |
| Fz |
| F4 |
| T3 |
| T4 |
| C3 |
| Cz |
| C4 |
| T5 |
| T6 |
| P3 |
| Pz |
| P4 |
| O1 |
| O2 |
| EO |

71=R   72=R   73=R   74=R   75=R   76=R   77=R

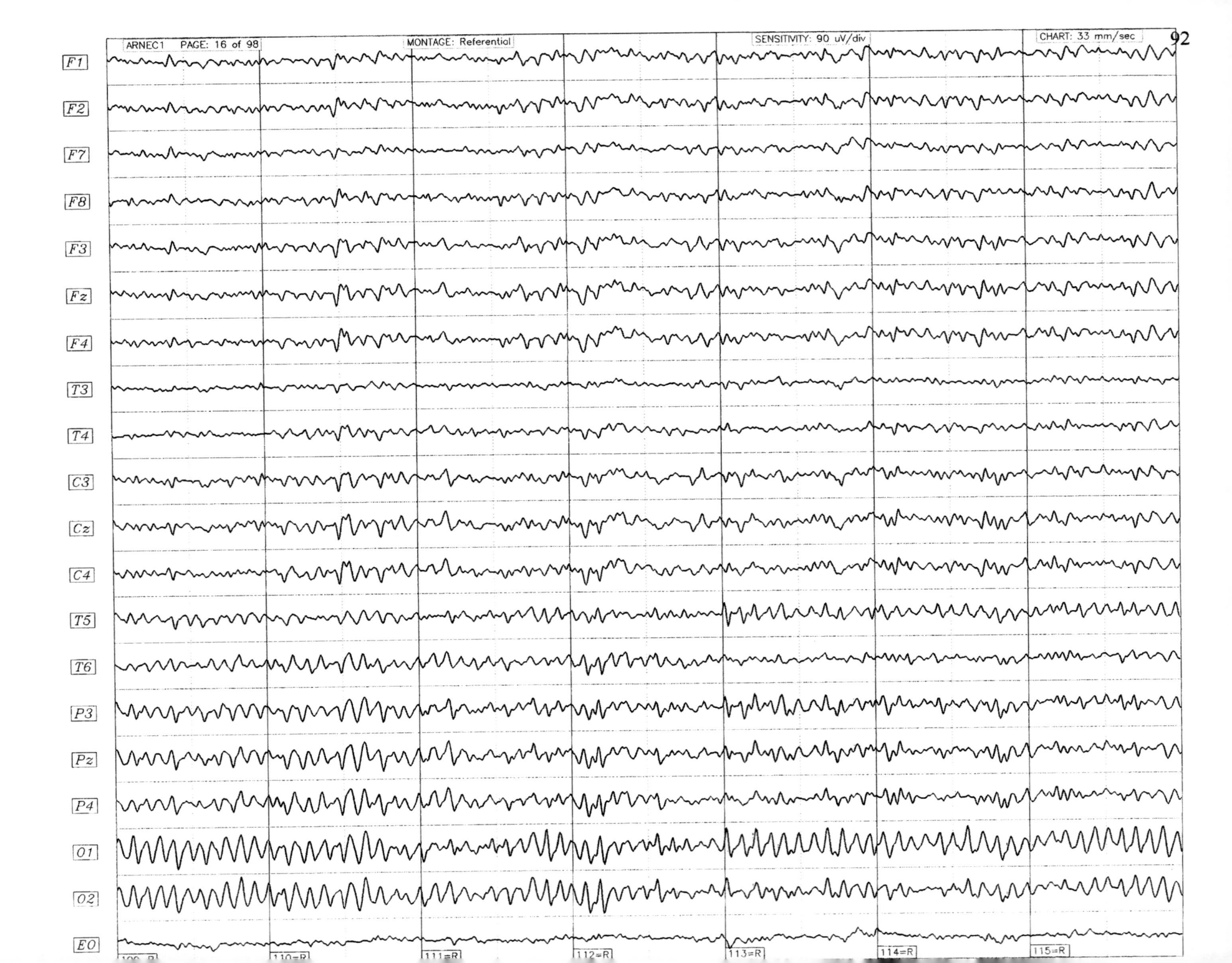

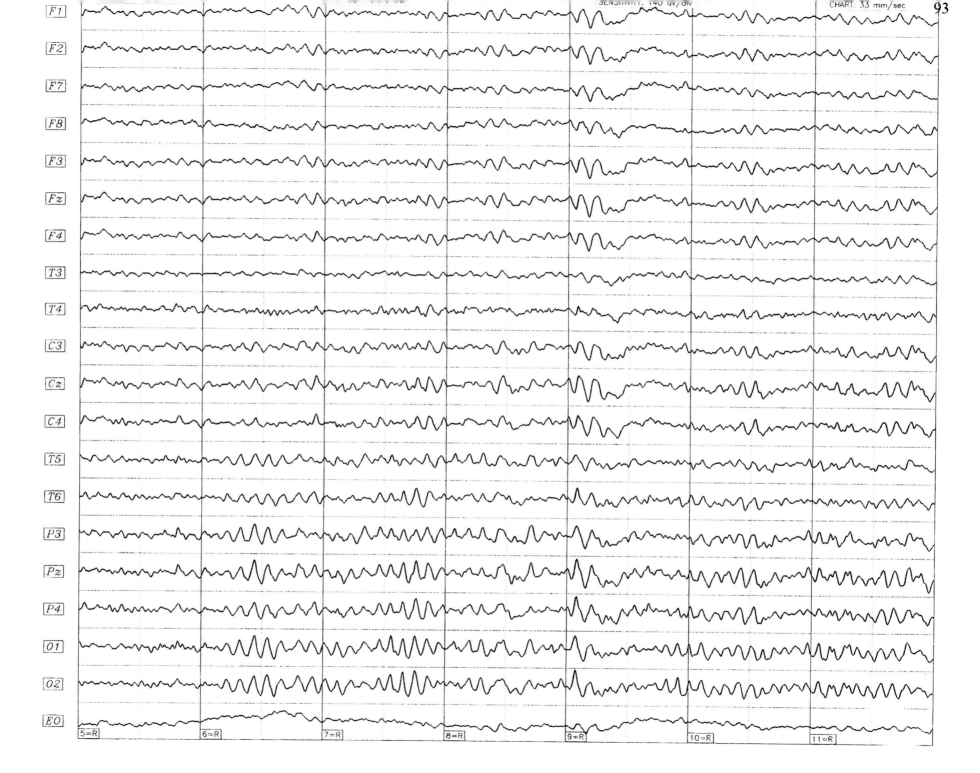

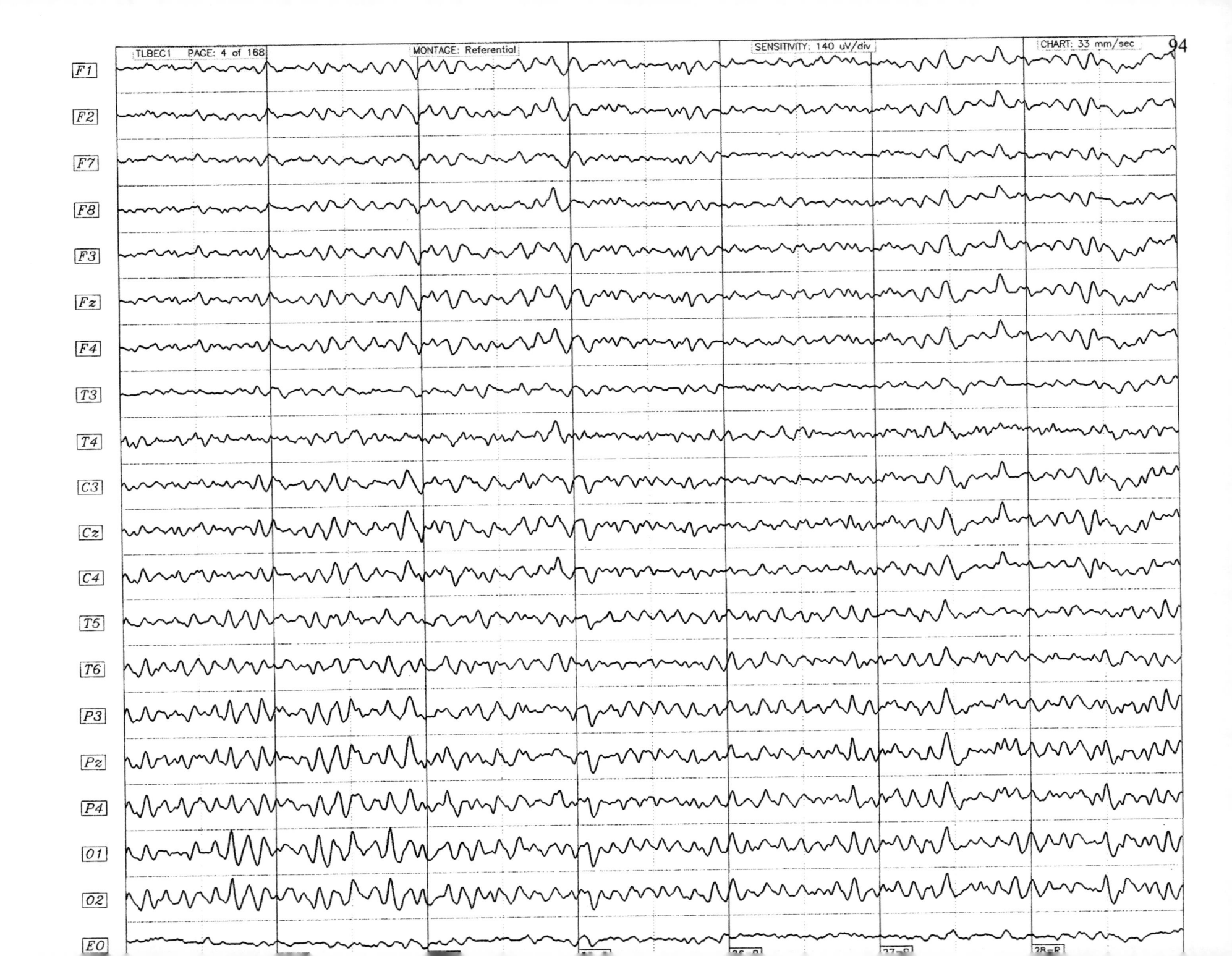

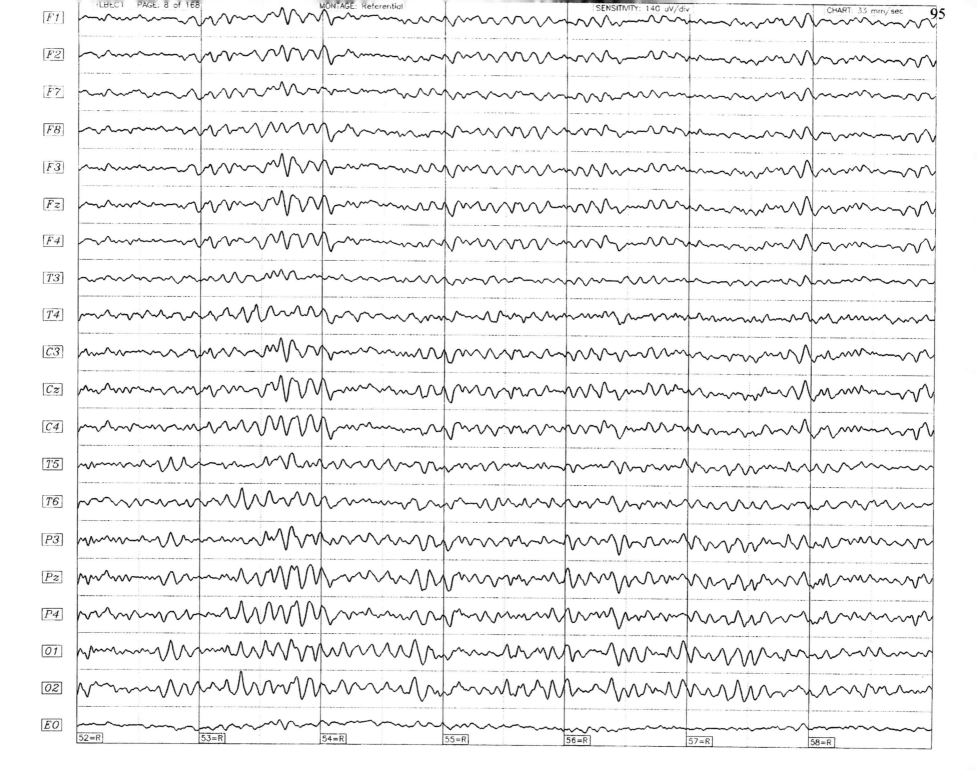

F1
F2
F7
F8
F3
Fz
F4
T3
T4
C3
Cz
C4
T5
T6
P3
Pz
P4
O1
O2
EO

52=R   53=R   54=R   55=R   56=R   57=R   58=R

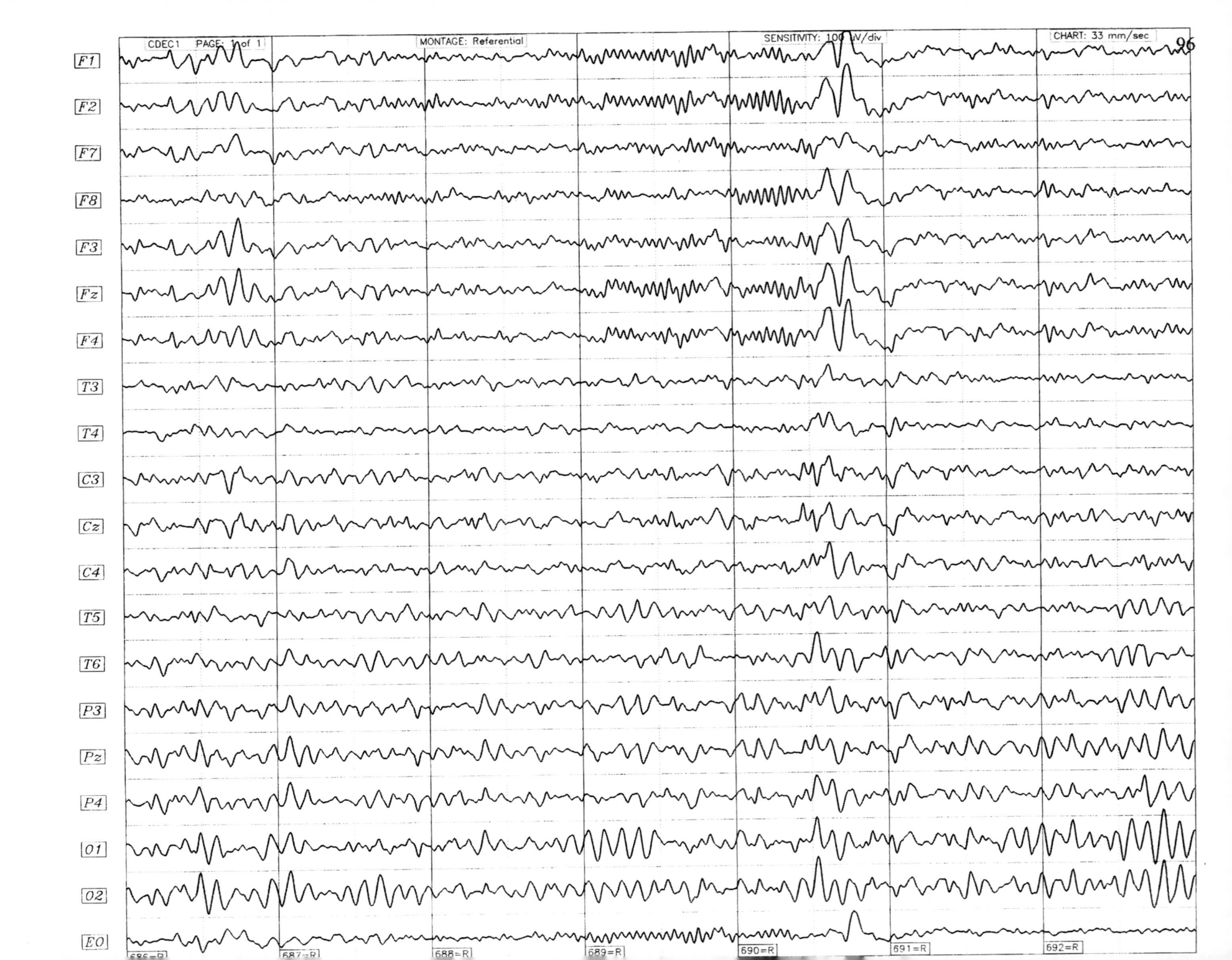

References

American Society of Electroneurodiagnostic Technologists, Inc. (1997). *Drugs & Their Effects on Neurodiagnostics.* Carroll, IA: ASET.

Bartel, P., Robinson, E., & Dium, W. (1995). Burst patterns occurring during drowsiness in clinical EEGs. *American Journal of EEG Technology,*:35, 283-295.

Bauer, G., & Bauer, R. (1999). EEG drug effects and central nervous system poisoning. In E. Niedermeyer & F. Lopes Da Silva (Eds.), *Electroencephalography: Basic principles, clinical applications, and related fields.* Baltimore: Williams & Wilkins, pp. 671-691.

Davidson, R. J. (1998a). Affective style and affective disorders: Perspectives from affective neuroscience. *Cognition & Emotion,*:12, 307-330.

Davidson, R. J. (1998b). Anterior electrophysiological asymmetries, emotion, and depression: Conceptual and methodological conundrums. *Psychophysiology*:35, 607-614.

Dement, W. (1999). The Promise of Sleep. New York: Dell. Duffy, F. H., Iyer, V. G., & Surwillo, W. W. (1989). *Clinical Electroencephalography and Topographic Brain Mapping: Technology and Practice.* New York: Springer-Verlag.

Fisch, B. J. (1991). *Spehlmann's EEG Primer* (2nd Edition). New York: Elsevier. 97

Glaze, D. G. (1990). Drug effects. In D. D. Daly & T. A. Pedley (Eds.), *Current Practice of Clinical Electroencephalography,* Second Edition. New York: Raven Press, pp. 489-512.

Goldensohn, E. S., Legatt, A. D., Koszer, S., & Wolf, S. M. (1998). *Goldensohn's EEG Interpretation: Problems of Overreading and Underreading (Second Revised and Updated Edition).*

Heller, W., Etienne, M. A., & Miller, G. A. (1995). Patterns of perceptual asymmetry in depression and anxiety: Implications for neuropsychological models of emotion and psychopathology. *Journal of Abnormal Psychology:* 104,327- 333.

Heller, W., Nitschke, J. B., Etienne, M. A., & Miller, G. A. (1997). Patterns of regional brain activity differentiate types of anxiety. *Journal of Abnormal Psychology:* 106(3), 376-385.

Hughes, J. (1994). *EEG in Clinical Practice (Second edition).* Boston: Butterworth-Heinemann.

Jaffe, R., & Brown, L. (1983). Tongue-movement artifacts in the electroencephalogram. *Clinical Electroencephalography:* 14(1), 57-59.

Klass, D. ,W. (1995), The continuing challenge of artifacts in the EEG, *American Journal of EEG Technology*: 35, 239-269.

Lee, S & Buchsbaum, M. S, (1987), Topographic mapping of EEG artifacts. *Clinical Electroencephalography*: 18,61-67.

Milnarich, R. F., Tourney, G., & Beckett, p, G. S, (1957), Electroencephalographic artifact arising from dentalrestorations. *Electroencephalography & Clinical Neurophysiology,*:~, 337-339.

Mowery, G. L. (1962). Artifacts. *American Journal of EEG Technology.* ~(2), 41-58.

O'Donnell, R. D., Berkhout, J., & Adey, W. R. (1974). Contamination of scalp EEG spectrum during contraction of cranio-facial muscles. *Electroencephalography & Clinical Neurophysiology.* 37, 145-151.

Oken, B. S. (1986). Filtering and aliasing of muscle activity in EEG frequency analysis. *Electroencephalography & Clinical Neurophysiology:* 64, 77-80.

Rosenfeld, J. P. (1997). EEG biofeedback of frontal alpha asymmetry in affective disorders. *Biofeedback:* 25(1), 8-25.

Santamaria, J., & Chiappa, K. H. (1987). The EEG of drowsiness in normal adults. *Journal of Clinical Neurophysiology:* 1, 327-382.

Westmoreland, B. F., Espinosa, R. E., & Klass, D. W. (1973). Significant prosopo-glosso-pharyngeal movements affecting the electroencephalogram. *American Journal of EEG Technology:~*, 59-70.

Wiedemann, G., Pauli, P., Dengler, W., Lutzenberger, W., Birbaumer, N., & Buckkremer, G. (1999). Frontal brain asymmetry as a biological substrate of emotions in patients with panic disorders. *Archives of General Psychiatry.* 56, 78- 84.

Wills, J., Nelson, A., Rice, J. & Black, F.W. (1993) The 98 Topoography of muscle activity in quantitative EEG. *Clinical Electroencephalography:* 24(3), 123-126.

Record # 22:
Epoch 38: Accept
Epoch 39: Accept
Epoch 40: Accept
Epoch 41: Accept
Epoch 42: Reject: eye movement, Fp1, Fp2, F7, F8, EO
Epoch 43: Reject: eye movement, Fp1, Fp2
Epoch 44: Reject: eye movement, Fp1, Fp2

Record # 23:
Epoch 45: Accept
Epoch 46: Reject: eye movement
Epoch 47: Accept
Epoch 48: Reject: eye movement, F7, F8, Fp1, Fp2, EO
Epoch 49: Accept
Epoch 50: Accept
Epoch 51: Reject: lateral eye movement (F7, F8). The event related potential is not greater than 50% above background, and so it would not be rejected due to it.

Record # 24:
Epoch 52: Accept
Epoch 53: Accept
Epoch 54: Reject: eye movement, especially on Fp1, Fp2
Epoch 55: Reject: lateral eye movement, F7, F8
Epoch 56: Reject: lateral eye movement, F7, F8, Fp1, Fp2

Epoch 57: Accept
Epoch 58: Reject: lateral eye movement.

Record # 25:
Epoch 59: Reject: lateral eye movement, F7, F8
Epoch 60: Reject: lateral eye movement, F7, F8
Epoch 61: Reject: lateral eye movement
Epoch 62: Reject: lateral eye movement
Epoch 63: Reject: eye movement
Epoch 64: Accept
Epoch 65: Accept

Record # 26:
Epoch 316: Reject: event related potential through center of epoch, and EMG on T3.
Epoch 317: Reject: EMG, T3
Epoch 318: Reject: event related potential near end of epoch on frontal channels; EMG on T3.
Epoch 319: Reject: EMG, T3; drowsiness seen in decreasing alpha amplitude and increased theta posteriorly.
Epoch 320: Reject: EMG and drowsiness.
Epoch 321: Reject: EMG and drowsiness.
Epoch 322: Reject: EMG and drowsiness.

Record # 27:

Epoch 323: Reject: EMG on T3 and drowsiness.
Epoch 324: Reject: EMG on T3
Epoch 325: Reject: EMG on T3
Epoch 326: Reject: EMG on T3, and event related potential about *1/3* into the epoch.
Epoch 327: Reject: EMG on T3
Epoch 328: Reject: EMG on T3
Epoch 329: Reject: EMG on T3

Record # 28:

Epoch 347: Reject: EMG on T3; eye movement.
Epoch 348: Reject: EMG and eye movement, Fp1, Fp2.
Epoch 349: Reject: EMG and eye movement, Fp1, Fp2
Epoch 350: Reject: EMG and eye movement.
Epoch 351: Reject: EMG, and drowsiness seen in posterior channels.
Epoch 352: Reject: EMG, drowsiness, and transient near end of epoch.
Epoch 353: Reject: EMG and transient early in epoch.

Record # 29:

Epoch 1: Accept
Epoch 2: Accept
Epoch 3: Accept
Epoch 4: Accept
Epoch 5: Reject: Event related potentials in last half a second.
Epoch 6: Accept
Epoch 7: Accept

Record # 30:

Epoch 8: Accept
Epoch 9: Accept
Epoch 10: Accept
Epoch 11: Accept
Epoch 12: Reject: eye movement, Fp1, Fp2, F7.
Epoch 13: Reject: eye movement, Fp1, Fp2, F7
Epoch 14: Reject: eye movement.

Record # 31:

Epoch 15: Accept
Epoch 16: Reject: eye movement, Fp1, Fp2, EO.
Epoch 17: Reject: eye movement
Epoch 18: Accept
Epoch 19: Accept
Epoch 20: Accept
Epoch 21: Accept

Record # 32:

Epoch 22: Reject: eye movement, EO, Fp1, Fp2
Epoch 23: Reject: eye movement.
Epoch 24: Reject: eye movement, EO, Fp1, Fp2
Epoch 25: Accept
Epoch 26: Reject: eye movement, EO, Fp1 , Fp2; the event related potential early in the epoch does not reach 50%.
Epoch 27: Accept
Epoch 28: Accept

Record # 33:

Epoch 29: Reject: eye movement, EO, Fp1, Fp2
Epoch 30: Accept
Epoch 31: Accept

Epoch 32: Reject: eye movement, EO, Fp1, Fp2
Epoch 33: Reject: eye movement, EO, Fp1, Fp2
Epoch 34: Accept
Epoch 35: Accept

Record # 34:
Epoch 36: Accept
Epoch 37: Reject: eye movement, EO, Fp1, Fp2
Epoch 38: Accept: event related potential does not reach 50% above background.
Epoch 39: Accept
Epoch 40: Reject: eye movement
Epoch 41: Reject: eye movement
Epoch 42: Accept

Record # 35:
Epoch 43: Accept
Epoch 44: Accept
Epoch 45: Reject: eye movement: EO,Fp1, Fp2
Epoch 46: Reject: eye movement, Fp1, Fp2
Epoch 47: Reject: eye movement, EO, Fp1, Fp2
Epoch 48: Accept
Epoch 49: Accept

Record # 36:
Epoch 50: Accept
Epoch 51: Accept
Epoch 52: Accept
Epoch 53: Accept
Epoch 54: Accept
Epoch 55: Accept
Epoch 56: Accept

Record # 37:
Epoch 57: Reject: event related potential just past the middle of the epoch.
Epoch 58: Accept
Epoch 59: Accept
Epoch 60: Reject: eye movement
Epoch 61: Reject: eye movement
Epoch 62: Accept
Epoch 63: Accept

Record # 38:
Epoch 64: Accept
Epoch 65: Accept
Epoch 66: Accept
Epoch 67: Reject: lateral eye movement, F7, F8, EO
Epoch 68: Reject: lateral eye movement, F7, F8
Epoch 69: Accept
Epoch 70: Accept

Record # 39:
Epoch 71: Accept
Epoch 72: Accept
Epoch 73: Accept
Epoch 74: Reject: eye movement
Epoch 75: Reject: eye movement, Fp1, Fp2, EO
Epoch 76: Accept
Epoch 77: Accept

Record # 40:
Epoch 78: Accept

Epoch 79: Accept
Epoch 80: Accept
Epoch 81 : Reject: eye movement: EO, Fp1, Fp2, F7
Epoch 82: Accept
Epoch 83: Reject: eye movement: EO, F7, F8, Fp1
Epoch 84: Reject: eye movement at beginning of epoch.

Record # 41:
Epoch 85: Accept
Epoch 86: Accept: ERP does not reach 50%.
Epoch 87: Accept
Epoch 88: Accept
Epoch 89: Reject: eye movement, EO, Fp1, Fp2
Epoch 90: Accept
Epoch 91: Reject: eye movement, EO, Fp1, Fp2

Record # 42:
Epoch 92: Reject: eye movement, EO, Fp1, Fp2
Epoch 93: Reject: eye movement, EO, Fp1, Fp2
Epoch 94: Reject: eye movement, EO, Fp1, Fp2
Epoch 95: Reject: eye movement
Epoch 96: Accept
Epoch 97: Accept
Epoch 98: Accept

Record # 43:
Epoch 106: Accept
Epoch 107: Accept
Epoch 108: Accept
Epoch 109: Accept
Epoch 110: Accept
Epoch 111: Reject: lateral eye movement, F7, F8, EO

Epoch 112: Accept

Record # 44:
Epoch 113: Accept
Epoch 114: Accept
Epoch 115: Accept
Epoch 116: Accept
Epoch 117: Reject: eye movement, EO, Fp1, Fp2
Epoch 118: Accept
Epoch 119: Accept

Record # 45:
Epoch 120: Reject: eye movement, EO, Fp1, Fp2
Epoch 121: Reject: eye movement, ERP.
Epoch 122: Accept
Epoch 123: Accept
Epoch 124: Accept
Epoch 125: Accept
Epoch 126: Reject: eye movement

Record # 46:
Epoch 134: Accept
Epoch 135: Accept
Epoch 136: Accept
Epoch 137: Accept
Epoch 138: Accept
Epoch 139: Accept
Epoch 140: Reject: eye movement

Record # 47:
Epoch 108: Accept

Epoch 109: Reject: eye movement and transient.
Epoch 110: Reject: event related potential
Epoch 111: Accept
Epoch 112: Accept
Epoch 113: Accept
Epoch 114: Reject: event related potential late in epoch.

Record # 48:
Epoch 115: Reject: eye movement, EO, Fp1, Fp2.
Epoch 116: Accept
Epoch 117: Accept
Epoch 118: Accept
Epoch 119: Accept
Epoch 120: Accept
Epoch 121: Accept

Record # 49:
Epoch 122: Accept
Epoch 123: Accept
Epoch 124: Accept
Epoch 125: Accept
Epoch 126: Accept
Epoch 127: Reject: small eye flutter
Epoch 128: Reject: event related potential late in epoch.

Record # 50:
Epoch 129: Accept
Epoch 130: Accept
Epoch 131: Accept
Epoch 132: Accept
Epoch 133: Accept
Epoch 134: Reject: transient

Epoch 135: Accept

Record # 51:
Epoch 136: Accept
Epoch 137: Accept
Epoch 138: Accept
Epoch 139: Accept
Epoch 140: Accept
Epoch 141: Accept
Epoch 142: Accept

Record # 52:
Epoch 143: Reject: event related potential.
Epoch 144: Reject: event related potential late in epoch.
Epoch 145: Accept
Epoch 146: Accept
Epoch 147: Reject: eye movement
Epoch 148: Accept
Epoch 149: Accept

Record # 53:
Epoch 150: Reject: eye movement
Epoch 151: Reject: eye movement
Epoch 152: Accept
Epoch 153: Reject: transient
Epoch 154: Reject: a paroxysmal transient that should be printed for evaluation, but rejected for qEEG data analysis.
Epoch 155: Reject: transient
Epoch 156: Reject: transient.

Record # 54:
Epoch 451: Reject: transient; T6 EMG.
Epoch 452: Reject: EMG, T6
Epoch 453: Reject: EMG, T6
Epoch 454: Accept
Epoch 455: Accept
Epoch 456: Reject: T3-T4 swaying in.
Epoch 457: Reject: T3-T4 sway; EMG, T6.

Record # 55:
Epoch 110: Accept
Epoch 111: Accept
Epoch 112: Accept
Epoch 113: Accept
Epoch 114: Accept
Epoch 115: Reject: lateral eye movement late in epoch, F7-F8.
Epoch 116: Reject: lateral eye movement, F7 -F8.

Record # 56:
Epoch 36: Accept
Epoch 37: Reject: drowsiness beginning with slowing of activity and
4 epochs later alpha flattens and there is more eye wandering.
Epoch 38: Reject: same reasons.
Epoch 39: Reject: lateral eye movement; drowsiness; ERP.
Epoch 40: Reject: lateral eye movement, F7-F8, and drowsiness. .
Epoch 41: Reject: lateral eye movement and drowsiness.
Epoch 42: Reject: lateral eye movement and drowsiness.

Record # 57:
Epoch 95: Reject: drowsiness or state change, 01, 02 with loss of
alpha definition.
Epoch 96: Reject: same reasons.

Epoch 97: Reject: same reasons.
Epoch 98: Reject: EMG, T3; ERD.
Epoch 99: Accept: ERP does not reach 50%.
Epoch 100: Accept
Epoch 101: Accept

Record # 58:
Epoch 112: Accept
Epoch 113: Accept
Epoch 114: Accept.
Epoch 115: Reject: state change.
Epoch 116: Reject: state change.
Epoch 117: Reject: state change.
Epoch 118: Accept

Record # 59:
Epoch 119: Accept
Epoch 120: Accept
Epoch 121: Accept
Epoch 123: Reject: transient.
Epoch 124: Reject: state change.
Epoch 125: Reject: state change.
Epoch 126: Accept

Record # 60:
Epoch 126: Accept
Epoch 127: Accept
Epoch 128: Accept
Epoch 129: Accept
Epoch 130: Reject: state change
Epoch 131: Accept
Epoch 132: Accept

Record # 61:
Epoch 154: Accept
Epoch 155: Accept: ERP's are less than 50%.
Epoch 156: Accept
Epoch 157: Accept
Epoch 158: Reject: state change.
Epoch 159: Reject: state change.
Epoch 160: Reject: state change.

Record # 62:
Epoch 34: Reject: EMG, T6; eye movement.
Epoch 35: Reject: EMG, T6; eye movement.
Epoch 36: Reject: eye movement, Fp1, Fp2, EO, F7, F8.
Epoch 37: Reject: eye movement; EMG, T6
Epoch 38: Reject: eye movement; EMG, T6
Epoch 39: Reject: eye movement; EMG, T6.
Epoch 40: Reject: EMG, T6.

Record # 63:
Epoch 41: Reject: EMG, T6
Epoch 42: Reject: EMG, T6
Epoch 43: Accept
Epoch 44: Reject: eye movement & ERP.
Epoch 45: Reject: eye movement, Fp1, Fp2, F7, F8, EO; EMG, T6.
Epoch 46: Reject: eye movement; EMG, T6.
Epoch 47: Reject: eye movement

Record # 64:
Epoch 71: Accept
Epoch 72: Accept

Epoch 73: Reject: EMG, T6
Epoch 74: Accept
Epoch 75: Reject: Sway in T3, T 4 which is of uncertain etiology (patient movement? electrodermal? cable movement? cap movement?); EMG, T6; possible state change, 01, 02.
Epoch 76: Reject: EMG, T6; sway, T3, T4;
Epoch 77: Reject: EMG, T6.

Record # 65:
Epoch 199: Accept
Epoch 200: Accept
Epoch 201: Accept
Epoch 202: Accept
Epoch 203: Accept
Epoch 204: Accept
Epoch 205: Accept

Record # 66:
Epoch 577: Reject: EMG, T6
Epoch 578: Reject: EMG, T6
Epoch 579: Accept
Epoch 580: Reject: EMG, T6
Epoch 581: Accept
Epoch 582: Accept
Epoch 583: Reject: EMG, T6

Record # 67:
Epoch 13: Reject: eye movement, Fp1, Fp2, EO; EMG,
Epoch 14: Reject: EMG, T3
Epoch 15: Reject: EMG, T3
Epoch 16: Reject: EMG, T3

Epoch 17: Reject: EMG, T3; eye movement, Fp1, Fp2,
Epoch 18: Reject: EMG, T3; eye movement, Fp1, Fp2, EO.
Epoch 19: Reject: EMG, T3; eye movement, Fp1, Fp2, EO.

Record # 68:
Epoch 54: Reject, EMG, T3; eye movement-EMG, Fp1, Fp2, F7. T3.
Epoch 55: Reject: EMG, T3.
Epoch 56: Reject: eye movement, Fp1, Fp2, EO; EMG,
Epoch 57: Reject: eye movement, Fp1, Fp2, EO.
Epoch 58: Reject: EMG, T3.
Epoch 59: Accept
Epoch 60: Accept

Record # 69:
Epoch 64: Reject: EMG, T3; transient in last half second.
Epoch 65: Reject: EMG, T3; transient.
Epoch 66: Reject: eye movement, Fp1, Fp2; EMG, T3?
Epoch 67: Reject: eye movement, Fp1, Fp2; EMG, T3?
Epoch 68: Reject: EMG, T3
Epoch 69: Reject: EMG, T3
Epoch 70: Reject: EMG, T3.

Record # 70:
Epoch 91: Reject: EMG, T3; eye movement, Fp1, Fp2.
Epoch 92: Accept
Epoch 93: Reject: lateral eye movement, F7, F8; EMG,
Epoch 94: Reject: lateral eye movement, F7, F8; EMG,
Epoch 95: Reject: EMG, T3
Epoch 96: Reject: EMG, T3; transient at end of epoch.
Epoch 97: Reject: EMG, T3; eye movement.

Record # 71:

Epoch 98: Reject: EMG, T3, F7; eye movement, Fp1, Fp2, EO, F7, F8. EO.
Epoch 99: Reject: EMG, T3.
Epoch 100: EMG, T3.
Epoch 101: Reject: EMG, T3
Epoch 102: Reject: EMG, T3
Epoch 103: Reject: EMG, T3
Epoch 104: Reject: EMG, T3; eye movement, Fp1, Fp2,

Record # 72:
Epoch 174: Reject: eye movement, Fp1, Fp2, EO.
Epoch 175: Reject: EMG, T4, T6, P4.
Epoch 176: Reject: eye movement; EMG.
Epoch 177: Reject: EMG, T3
Epoch 178: Reject: EMG, T3 and frontally; eye movement.
Epoch 179: Reject: eye movement, Fp1, Fp2; EMG frontally and T3.
Epoch 180: Reject: eye movement, Fp1, Fp2, EO; EMG.

Record # 73:
Epoch 488: Reject: EMG, Fp1, Fp2, T3.
Epoch 489: Accept
Epoch 490: Accept
Epoch 491: Reject: transient.
Epoch 492: Reject: EMG, T3 and frontally; eye movement, Fp1, Fp2, EO.
Epoch 493: Reject: EMG, T3 and frontally; eye movement, Fp1, Fp2, EO.
Epoch 494: Accept

Record # 74:
Epoch 498: Accept
Epoch 499: Accept

Epoch 500: Reject: eye movement at end of epoch, Fp1, Fp2, EO.
Epoch 501: Reject: eye movement at beginning of epoch, Fp1, Fp2, EO.
Epoch 502: Reject: eye movement
Epoch 503: Reject: eye movement, Fp1, Fp2, EO.
Epoch 504: Reject: eye movement, Fp1, Fp2, EO.

Record # 75:
Epoch 134: Reject: state change/state change.
Epoch 135: Reject: transient.
Epoch 136: Reject: EMG frontally; state change.
Epoch 137: Reject: state change.
Epoch 138: Reject: event related potential in mid-epoch.
Epoch 139: Reject: state change.
Epoch 140: Reject: eye movement at end of epoch.

Record # 76:
Epoch 155: Reject: state change; transient mid-epoch.
Epoch 156: Reject: eye movement, Fp1, Fp2, EO.
Epoch 157: Reject: eye movement, Fp1, Fp2, EO.
Epoch 158: Accept
Epoch 159: Reject: transient/event related potential.
Epoch 160: Accept
Epoch 161: Accept

Record # 77:
Epoch 162: Accept
Epoch 163: Accept
Epoch 164: Reject: state change.
Epoch 165: Reject: state change.
Epoch 166: Reject: possible state change.

Epoch 167: Reject: state change.
Epoch 168: Reject: state change.

Record # 78:
Epoch 3: Reject: state change/state change.
Epoch 4: Accept
Epoch 5: Reject: lateral eye movement, F7, F8.
Epoch 6: Reject: lateral eye movement, F7, F8, EO.
Epoch 7: Reject: lateral eye movement, F7, F8, EO.
Epoch 8: Accept
Epoch 9: Reject: lateral eye movement, F7, F8, EO.

Record # 79:
Epoch 10: Accept
Epoch 11: Accept
Epoch 12: Reject: eye movement.
Epoch 13: Accept
Epoch 14: Accept
Epoch 15: Accept
Epoch 16: Reject: lateral eye movement, F7, F8.

Record # 80:
Epoch 17: Accept
Epoch 18: Reject: eye movement, Fp1, Fp2, F7, F8, EO.
Epoch 19: Reject: eye movement
Epoch 20: Accept
Epoch 21: Reject: drowsiness, alpha diminishing.
Epoch 22: Reject: drowsiness.
Epoch 23: Reject: drowsiness.

Record # 81:
Epoch 24: Accept

Epoch 25: Accept
Epoch 26: Reject: state change/drowsiness
Epoch 27: Reject: state change/drowsiness
Epoch 28: Reject: state change/drowsiness
Epoch 29: Reject: state change/drowsiness
Epoch 30: Reject: state change/drowsiness

Record # 82:
Epoch 31: Reject: lateral eye movement, F7, F8, EO.
Epoch 32: Reject: lateral eye movement, F7, F8, EO.
Epoch 33: Reject: lateral eye movement, F7, F8, EO.
Epoch 34: Accept
Epoch 35: Accept
Epoch 36: Accept
Epoch 37: Reject: eye movement

Record # 83:
Epoch 38: Reject: eye movement
Epoch 39: Reject: eye movement
Epoch 40: Accept
Epoch 41: Accept
Epoch 42: Reject: eye movement, F7, F8.
Epoch 43: Reject: eye movement
Epoch 44: Reject: eye movement

Record # 84:
Epoch 45: Reject: lateral eye movement, F7, F8, EO.
Epoch 46: Reject: lateral eye movement.
Epoch 47: Reject: eye movement.
Epoch 48: Accept
Epoch 49: Accept
Epoch 50: Accept

Epoch 51: Accept

Record # 85:
Epoch 52: Accept
Epoch 53: Accept
Epoch 54: Accept
Epoch 55: Reject: eye movement, Fp1, Fp2, F7, F8, EO; EMG, F8.
Epoch 56: Reject: lateral eye movement, F7, F8, EO; EMG, F8.
Epoch 57: Reject: lateral eye movement, F7, F8, EO.
Epoch 58: Accept

Record # 86:
Epoch 59: Accept
Epoch 60: Reject: EMG, Fp1, Fp2, F7, F8.
Epoch 61: Reject: frontal EMG; eye movement.
Epoch 62: Reject: eye movement, Fp1, Fp2, F7, EO;
Epoch 63: Reject: EMG, Fp1, Fp2, F7, F8.
Epoch 64: Accept
Epoch 65: Reject: transients.

Record # 87:
Epoch 67: Accept
Epoch 68: Accept
Epoch 69: Reject: transient.
Epoch 70: Reject: transient.
Epoch 71: Accept
Epoch 72: Accept
Epoch 73: Your authors disagree: Jay accepts; Cory rejects, perceiving the decrease in 01 and 02 alpha and increase in central-frontal alpha, which continues into epoch 74 on the next Record #, as possible drowsiness.

Record # 88:
Epoch 74: Reject: eye movement
Epoch 75: Accept
Epoch 76: Accept
Epoch 77: Reject: lateral eye movement, F7, F8.
Epoch 78: Reject: lateral eye movement, F7, F8.
Epoch 79: Accept
Epoch 80: Accept

Record # 89:
Epoch 110: Reject: lateral eye movement, F7, F8.
Epoch 111: Reject: lateral eye movement, F7, F8.
Epoch 112: Accept
Epoch 113: Accept
Epoch 114: Accept
Epoch 115: Accept
Epoch 116: Accept

Record # 90:
Epoch 46: Reject: eye movement, Fp1, Fp2, EO; transient.
Epoch 47: Accept
Epoch 48: Reject: eye movement.
Epoch 49: Reject: eye movement.
Epoch 50: Reject: eye movement.
Epoch 51: Reject: eye movement.
Epoch 52: Accept

Record # 91:
Epoch 71: Reject: eye movement, Fp1, Fp2.
Epoch 72: Accept
Epoch 73: Accept
Epoch 74: Reject: event related potential, mid-epoch.

Epoch 75: Accept
Epoch 76: Accept
Epoch 77: Reject: eye movement, Fp1, Fp2, F7, F8, EO.

Record # 92:
Epoch 109: Accept
Epoch 110: Reject: event related potential, mid-epoch.
Epoch 111: Accept
Epoch 112: Accept
Epoch 113: Reject: event related potential, late in epoch; eye movement.
Epoch 114: Accept
Epoch 115: Accept

Record # 93:
Epoch 5: Accept: appears desynchronized rather than drowsy.
Epoch 6: Reject: lateral eye movement, F7, F8.
Epoch 7: Accept
Epoch 8: Reject: transient.
Epoch 9: Reject: transient.
Epoch 10: Accept
Epoch 11: Reject: transient begins at the end of epoch.

Record # 94:
Epoch 22: Reject: eye movement
Epoch 23: Accept
Epoch 24: Reject: event related potential
Epoch 25: Accept
Epoch 26: Accept
Epoch 27: Reject: event related potential, mid-epoch.
Epoch 28: Reject: slow transient.

Record # 95:

Epoch 52: Reject: state change.

Epoch 53: Reject: transient

Epoch 54: Reject: transient

Epoch 55: Accept

Epoch 56: Accept

Epoch 57: Reject: transient

Epoch 58: Reject: state change.

Record # 96:

Epoch 686: Accept

Epoch 687: Accept

Epoch 688: Accept

Epoch 689: Reject: transient and beta spindles.

Epoch 690: Reject: transient and beta spindling.

Epoch 691: Reject: transient

Epoch 692: Accept